Every Woman's Guide to
Beautiful Hair
at Any Age

LEARN WHAT CAN BE DONE TO KEEP A
BEAUTIFUL HEAD OF HAIR FOR A LIFETIME

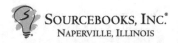
SOURCEBOOKS, INC.®
NAPERVILLE, ILLINOIS

LISA AKBARI

Published by Sourcebooks, Inc.
P.O. Box 4410, Naperville, Illinois 60567-4410
(630) 961-3900
FAX: (630) 961-2168
www.sourcebooks.com

Library of Congress Cataloging-in-Publication Data

Akbari, Lisa.
  Every woman's guide to beautiful hair at any age : learn what can be done to keep a beautiful head of hair for a lifetime / Lisa Akbari.
    p. cm.
  ISBN-13: 978-1-4022-0877-5
  ISBN-10: 1-4022-0877-4
  1. Hair--Care and hygiene. 2. Beauty, Personal. 3. Women--Health and hygiene. I. Title.
  RL91.A33 2007
  646.7'24--dc22

                          2007035310

                   Printed and bound in Canada
                   WC 10 9 8 7 6 5 4 3 2 1

Every Woman's Guide to Beautiful Hair at Any Age

LEARN WHAT CAN BE DONE TO KEEP A BEAUTIFUL HEAD OF HAIR FOR A LIFETIME

DEDICATION

I dedicate this book first to my soul mate, my friend, my husband, Hooshang Akbari, for thirty years of allowing me to "Do Me." To my two blessings and truly gifts from God, my daughters Raumesh and Raumina Akbari, for definitely being the loving positive energy and source of motivation in my life.

To my mother Clara Macklin for precisely, completely, and without distrust being the essence of a strong mother and woman. To my brother Tommie Macklin, who has made a commitment to stay and help fulfill the vision.

ACKNOWLEDGMENTS

Thanks to my agent Marlene for helping me to see what was right in front of me.

Thanks to my editor Deb Werksman for always challenging me.

And a special thanks to my family, friends, patients, students, and colleagues for all their support and encouragement.

I must acknowledge, as I have recognized, that there is a power higher than I that allows my point of view. This acceptance authorizes my soul to boast appreciation. This book and all the knowledge and power that are given to me to realize my mission, sanction me to give tribute to my own personal higher power, my Lord and my Savior, Jesus Christ. To God be the glory.

CONTENTS

INTRODUCTION

Before writing this book, I thought a lot about women and their hair because I wanted to get to the root of the problems of hair. I thought that in many ways women would be better off if God had never given us hair at all. The reason for such a radical thought is that, if we did not have hair, then we would not have to worry about it. Think about how much wasted money, drama, and even trauma this—our crowning glory—has caused. Women, on average, spend $1,200 a year on their hair, which does not include the extras, whereas men spend on average $250 a year, which does include extras.

Women also have a lot of drama surrounding their hair. For example, if a black woman straightens her curly hair, she may be thought to be denying her ethnicity by trying to be like someone she is not. If a white woman perms her straight hair, she is often accused of looking too ethnic. These are just two examples of cultural expectations surrounding women and their hair. Everyone has an opinion about how a woman should wear her hair, and many women believe they must take into account what others think in order to be accepted. In other words, women are expected to appear a certain way and stay in their place, even when it comes to hair.

In order to achieve this expected look, women abuse, misuse, bully, and damage their hair as they manipulate it into shape, all of which ages their hair. Sadly, the joy of the look is short-lived, and many women still are not happy. All the money, time, drama, and trauma spent on this arduous process of manipulation causes many women to suffer from what I call *hair depression*, because the tragic reality is that there are a number of women who are just simply depressed about their hair.

I believe that one of the big reasons why we women deal with hair trauma and drama and suffer from hair depression is that many of us have not learned to accept, respect, appreciate, and understand our hair in its natural state.

Well, ladies, it is time to take a ride on the hair freedom train. It should always be your choice to wear your hair naturally, chemically altered, or any other way you want. But you must first stop placing value on what someone else thinks about your hair and stop making choices to alter the style of your hair before becoming educated about that choice.

Real Freedom Begins within Our Minds

My prayer and hope is that this book will facilitate the process of solving a problem that we have made bigger than it ever should have become. Your hair is truly your crown. It covers and protects your head from the environment, while providing the image of yourself that you want to project to the world. But what happens when you age? What happens when your hair ages?

My primary mission is to help women solve their hair problems. This book is out to convince women that, no matter what age you are or what changes you are going through, all you need to do is just take better care of your hair and scalp, and everything will be okay. All I want is a way to make women understand how easy it is to stop hair challenges, and that is just what *Every Woman's Guide to Beautiful Hair at Any Age* is meant to do for you.

What Is Aging Hair?

How can hair age? How can the scalp age? Well, *to age* means to become old, grow old, get older. Aging hair and scalp mean just that. Your hair grows in its own life cycles, and within each life cycle your hair can grow old and even die before its time. When we think about getting older, we perhaps think about our body becoming weaker, more fragile, and not looking and feeling as vibrant as it did when we were younger. But we know that if we stop and put together a plan of health, eating right, exercising, and just taking care to have a nutritionally sound body, mind, and spirit, we won't become weak and fragile, and die before our time. The thrust of this book is not to talk about what happens to our body as it ages, but to discuss our hair as it ages. My purpose is to help you come to understand and know that you are free, truly free, to choose how you wear your hair. Free to make a choice as a woman with curly hair to wear it chemically straightened and as a woman with straight hair to wear it chemically curled, without it some-how meaning that you are assimilating or selling out. You will learn how to keep your hair young and vibrant even with changes, natural or chemical, at any age throughout your life, as well as throughout your hair's life cycles.

We expect our hair to start graying as we age, and most of us can accept gray hair, or we know what to do about it if we can't. But we wonder what our hair might look like when we approach the menopausal stage; we all fear the day when our hair might start thin-ning. What can we do then? Studies have shown that thinning hair is one of the biggest mysteries and concerns connected with aging. After reading this guide, you will understand hair thinning and how you can stop the most common type of thinning. You may be surprised to learn that what you thought was an uncontrollable thinning of the strand can actually be controlled. I want to show you how you can eliminate and even prevent this negative aging process. What you learn from this book will teach you how to keep your hair and scalp looking younger until the hair completes all of its life cycles. You can become proactive and not just reactive as it relates to your hair and scalp's aging. Your hair and scalp can look, feel, and remain young now and for years to come.

Aging Hair Defined

An aging hair strand is dehydrated, weak, fragile, and thin, and it will die before its time. Many women have hair that is aging faster than they are. Before reading this guide, you have probably asked yourself the question, "Why read a book on aging hair?" Some of you may have been curious, but most of you, I suspect, needed and wanted help, because you have hair issues or perhaps have been dealing with some level of hair crisis most of your life. Now that you are getting older, you may feel a sense of urgency because most believe that aging means suffering with some level of hair loss. So, if you want help, help is here! But help is here only if you read with an open mind. Don't look for any magic, cure-all, special ointments, potions, or concoctions (although I do recommend my personally made products, which are safe, reliable, very effective, and extremely beneficial). I take a different point of view, that of empowering with knowledge.

My view derives from counseling and from treating the hair of thousands of women, as well as from the many studies that I have conducted to prove my theories about why women lose hair. This guide is about approaching hairstyling, not as a way to style some fibers and make them look pretty, but as a way of caring for your hair as an important appendage of the scalp. Thinking about it this way makes you realize that your hair is a living part of you!

You may be thinking, "Is hair that serious? Do I need to get that deep with it?" The answer is yes. Hair, although a dead substance, is so important to us that it seems to take on its own life.

Our hair has the ability to determine and dictate our mood. The good news is that you can personally stop the negative aging process of your hair and scalp. I understand what you are going through, and I will enlighten you to view your hair in a way that you have never viewed your hair and scalp before. Many of you have looked at your hair and thought that now that you are getting older, it is time for your hair to get older, and you just have to accept aging hair as a fact of life. But I am here to tell you that you do not have to accept it! You can change the so-called "predetermined outcome" because you can take control and change what seems inevitable, by building a special relationship with your hair, in order to stop damaging your hair.

Chapter One:

What's Happening to My Hair?

"Age is a question of mind over matter.
If you don't mind, it doesn't matter."
—Satchel Paige

...or does it?

In this chapter, you will learn about how your personality relates to your hair and about how personal life challenges and changes as you age can lead to decisions about how you treat your hair. And those decisions all too often lead to choices that age your hair. This makes you personally responsible. For instance, you may do things that seem harmless. Sometimes you just want to feel better about yourself; sometimes you may feel that you must fit into whatever season of life that you are in at that time; sometimes you may just want a change. The problem is that some of those reasons, because they are not well thought out, can prompt you to do things to your hair that cause aging damage.

First, we must agree that how we behave in certain situations will determine what happens down the road. Understanding this will supply wisdom that will help you stop and think before you act, so you pay attention when your mind sends up red flags. Think for a minute about when you've had most of your hair tribulations. Something within you was the core cause, and that something was part of your personality, which determines behavior. Now, I am not implying that all of your hair problems are caused by your behavior, but studies do show that hair breakage, some scalp disorders, and even some forms of balding (alopecia) stem from neglect, abuse, and poor hair and scalp care habits and choices. We seem to be faced with many of these things, and they occur more and more as we age. I am aware that there are causes for some hair and scalp problems that are beyond your control, but let's stick for now to the things you can control.

Over the years, some have grouped all hair and scalp problems into one pile, and blamed all of their problems on anything and anybody other than themselves. However, there are ways that you personally can take charge and avoid many hair tribulations. The number one thing that you will need to do is make adjustments in your behavior, taking control of the actions or things that occur as they relate to your hair. There are consequences for the spur-of-the-moment decisions that we make. We may pay for them with hair damage. Understand that I am not here to take the spontaneity out of your life and leave you with boring hair. I am actually going to teach you how to fulfill all the hair whims you can dream up; most importantly, I am going to empower you to care for your hair safely, without aging it. By policing your behavior, you will have young, vibrant hair with style at any age. The number one thing that I hear from the women I counsel is that, during the time of their hair problems, all they did was simply go into a salon one day, ask for something specific, and come out with something totally different from what they had requested. In other words, they shifted the blame for their hair problems to their stylists. I am aware that many stylists make mistakes, and the clients pay and suffer dearly for them. However, you have more control than you think concerning your salon visits, as well as other situations during hair calamities. Once you recognize what you can do to gain control of the situation, you will lessen your hair problems, and you will be on your way to understanding how to be in charge of almost every hair situation; gaining control will stop the premature aging of your hair.

How Did I Learn to Help?

I came up with my conclusions after being in the hair industry for over thirty years, working on the salon side of the industry first, as a hairstylist, doing all the hands-on styling, cutting, and coloring. Now I am a trichologist, researching, conducting studies on, writing about, and analyzing hair. Year after year, I have watched clients grapple with the same hair problems over and over, in a never-ending cycle. Many women just don't "get it," and, early on, neither did I.

Back in my styling days, I could not understand why some of my clients seemed to have more hair and scalp problems than others. I thought, "It must be stress, nerves, diet, and we must not forget the most popular reason, age. Surely getting older must have something to do with my clients' hair problems." Of course, all of the things that I mentioned can play a role, because the overall health and balance of the body can sometimes establish how healthy your hair grows. But the mere mention of your health when talking about hair will get clients off on the wrong track, because there are so many factors to consider when evaluating one's overall health. But I found many very healthy people with very unhealthy hair.

So, as I looked at the people who put the care of their hair in my hands, I began to take a close look at everything, and I went on a mission to fix everything. I put together the best hair and scalp care program for each individual who came through my door. I started with a full hair and scalp analysis and in-clinic treatments to stabilize any hair problems. Once the problem was stable, I put together a home hair care program and additional counseling for her as well as her regular stylist. I recommended regular follow-up examinations and treatments to ensure that she was on the right track for maintenance and prevention. Unfortunately, my program worked for some, but not for others, and some of the ones it did work for seemed to encounter a setback or two after awhile. I found myself in a situation where I did not understand what was going on and what to do. Believe me, I have been there before, as I tried many times to conquer the hair tribulations of women. I said to myself, "There must be something more. I must be overlooking something." Then I realized I was trying to fix a problem that was not solely my problem to fix. I needed to involve the client in a way that I had not done before. So I began to notice and record the things that were said about the times surrounding the hair problems. I also looked at what was going on in the client's life at the time of the hair setback.

Finally, I began to compare the various behaviors.

I found that when a client was going through a challenge in her life, a certain level of neglect in hair and scalp care was apparent. Most of these cases involved a life-altering change, such as a divorce, a new job, a new boyfriend, or becoming a mom. My client would express that she needed to or felt forced to change things about the way she looked. It is as if your hair just goes along with all your whims, kicking and screaming, trying to hold on by a single thread. Or shall I say by a single hair? Depending on the situation, the change may be subtle or drastic, anything from a simple haircut to a permanent straightener or wave. There is nothing wrong with change; there are many times when change is good. Here I am talking about impromptu, hasty changes that ended up causing aging damage to your hair and scalp. Let me give you an example. You may have said, "I need to change my hair color. I look too drab with the one I have." Or you might have said, "I want my curly hair straight," or "I want my straight hair curly." When you end up with hair or scalp damage, you proceed to blame something as variable as stress. You must recognize and analyze the hair change before making it, looking at all the pros and cons. This is important so that you don't damage your hair and scalp in the process of making the change.

I want you to get the look you desire, while behaving as you should. You may ask, "How?" First, stop being a victim and stop letting others talk you into doing things to your hair without your first knowing everything you need to know in order to keep your hair and scalp safe. Second, stop asking for things to be done to your hair just because it feels right or is fashionable. Third, understand that an ounce of prevention is worth a pound of cure, especially as it relates to your hair and scalp. Finally, remember that education is power; the more you know before you act, the more control you will have over your hair situations. All these things will help you behave as you should, as it relates to your hair, while concurrently influencing others to behave as they should. I guarantee that you will see a difference in how healthy and full of life your hair will be in each and every one of its cycles of life.

Before Making the Hair Change

Before changing your hair in any way, first ask yourself some simple questions, and do an overall self-examination.

1. Why am I making a hair change?
2. Are my hair and scalp ready to survive the new changes?
3. Is this hair change really what I want, or do I feel forced?
4. Is this change safe?
5. How will this change affect my hair and scalp?
6. If I don't like the change, am I willing to stay with the change until my hair and scalp are ready for a "change back" or yet another change?
7. Have I found the correct hair care professionals for my change?
8. Will this hair change cause me to become stressed out?
9. Can I take care of this change?
10. Am I willing to follow a strict hair and scalp care program after the change?
11. Is this something that I really want to do?

If after answering the questions above, you decide to make this hair change, then it is time for the next step. Do your research, which will include finding the right professional to help with the change. If you research and find that there are too many risks involved or that you can't find the right professional, then do not behave negatively (do not make the change anyway).

Here's an example of a chemical service and a checklist for research questions. I think it will be appropriate to use a chemical hair service as our example because permanent waves (perms), relaxers, and coloring are the leading causes of hair and scalp damage and hair loss among women.

Research Questions
1. Which chemicals will be used?
2. What are the dangers of using those chemicals?
3. What effects will the chemicals have on my hair type?
4. What percentage of hair loss occurs when these chemicals are used on a hair type such as mine?
5. What should I expect the outcome to be?
6. How often can I safely use these chemicals?

Once you have researched as much as you can about the chemicals, you should start researching professional help.
1. Who has experience working with this type of chemical service on my hair type?
2. Can he or she answer the questions I have about the chemicals?
3. Can I talk with some of his or her clients who have received this chemical service and who have my hair type? (If possible,

arrange a meeting with them in person, or perhaps try a phone appointment.)

4. Is a maintenance hair and scalp program offered? What needs to be done for proper upkeep?

By doing this legwork beforehand, you will be less likely to have problems afterward. As you become educated and follow the steps laid out in this guide, you will be ready to make any hair change.

Preventing Aging of Your Hair and Scalp

When life challenges and changes occur that seem to overcrowd our schedule, we go into automatic pilot mode. We instantly start prioritizing our life, trimming off things we think are not important or can wait, and doing things in a way that will help us save time (that is, cutting corners). We justify this by telling ourselves that it's only because we are busy, and as soon as things settle down, we are going to get back to the things that we need to do for ourselves. Believe me, I have done it, we all have done it, but that does not make it right. The problem is that, in many cases when you go into this type of mode, something suffers. What you are really saying is, "I will have a healthy head of hair only when it fits into my schedule." Before you know it, in order to get things done, you do things in a shortcut fashion or do not do them at all. In the course of it all, you tend to neglect the care of your hair and scalp. We may not walk out of the house with our hair styled in a mess, but we will walk out the house with our scalp and hair care in a mess.

Let me explain what I mean with an example. Think about your to-do list. You went to the salon and had your hair shampooed and styled; now you check that off your list. You have every intention of shampooing and conditioning your hair later this week, but as the days go by, you still have not shampooed. You look in the mirror and say, "My hair does not look too bad; maybe if I use hairspray or my curling iron just to touch up the style, I can get by." But as I said earlier, something does suffer. You took the time to curl your dirty hair, but you did not take the time to shampoo and condition it. That's my point about style versus care: style in place, but scalp and hair dirty. Now I know you may be thinking, "What choice do I have?" You did what you had time to do, and you are doing the best you can, but that does not make it right. Your behavior will cause aging damage to your hair and scalp sooner than later. I don't agree with you when you say that you are doing the best you can, but I do believe that you are doing the best that you know how to do. You must learn better so that you will do better. Let's face it: if you have time to take a shower, you have time to shampoo and condition your hair. In this book, I will give you many steps to prevent aging your hair and scalp. You will learn quick-fix styles that are safe and that will do more than just get you by. Learning these styles will empower you to never again sacrifice the care of your hair and scalp because you "don't have time."

Take the Time

I remember a particular situation when one of my clients still complained about hair dryness a week after I gave her a regimen to follow that should have solved her dry hair problems. After a short talk, I realized that she had never followed my simple instructions. I asked her why, and her answer was, and I quote her, "I did not have the time." As I touched her dehydrated hair, I asked her, "Then why bother? Why waste your time looking for a solution when you are not going to take the time to learn how to follow the steps?"

If you are willing to stop and make the proper adjustments in your behavior, I believe that you will have a wonderful and safe relationship with your hair. You will be able to make a choice to make any change you like, because the changes you make will be the ones that are right for your hair and scalp. No more impromptu, remiss choices, and no more aging damage to your hair and scalp. You can do this.

CHAPTER TWO:

DOES AGING AFFECT MY HAIR?

From puberty to menopause, your hair will change as you age, but not as much as you might think, and not the way you might think. Do you just sit back and watch the aging process, or can you control or change how your hair and scalp age? In this chapter, you will learn what happens, as well as why and how it happens.

The Facts about Aging Damage

Puberty usually starts between the ages of 8 and 14. As girls approach this time of their lives, hair becomes a big part of how they express themselves. Many girls begin to experiment with new cuts and styles, as well as with the latest hair products and chemicals that promise beautiful hair. Some girls experience hair and scalp damage in the process. This damage is most likely their first experience with aging hair, even at that young age.

Menopause usually happens in a woman's life between the ages of 45 and 60. As a woman approaches this period, many things change within her body; her hair and skin will change, and the needs of her hair and scalp become even greater. Studies have shown that, as we grow older, hair growth slows down and our skin loses its natural moisture. Your hair experiences some natural changes as you grow older, such as in color or texture, as new hair is cycled in. But as a result of aging damage, many of the changes you may think are natural are not. For example, a coarse strand can become thin as the hair strand itself ages, but it can also become thin unnaturally from premature aging damage from chemicals or overdrying. However, hair, unlike the human body, can and will replace itself. When you damage your hair strands beyond repair, and the hairs die away, new hair will grow in, ready to replace what was just killed off. What a blessing! Some women believe that once the hair strand is damaged, it is and always will be damaged, but that simply is not true.

I have interviewed many women who feel certain that the hair damage that they experienced as girls has, as some have phrased it, "stunted future hair growth." I think it is important that we discuss the likelihood of this being true, due to the number of women who believe this misconception.

Hair shaft (strand) damage can be permanent to that particular strand, but it is not permanent to the new strands that will grow from your scalp thereafter. The head of hair that you had at age 10 is not still on your head at age 45. Your hair grows and sheds in cycles, and the complete life of each strand is no more than six years in length. I will talk more about the hair growth cycle later in this book.

Any hair that was damaged as you went through puberty is no longer with you. The reason why so many women have long histories of hair problems, often spanning throughout most of their lives, is, quite simply, because of a history of poor habits throughout life. After conducting countless studies to find out why women are losing their hair unnecessarily, I found one thing that seems to be constant: many with similar hair and scalp problems had similar hair care habits and regimens passed along to them. Many of us get our hair care habits from whomever we grew up around: our moms, aunts, big sisters, and so on. Whatever we saw them do to their hair, we tried to do the same. So we ended up with some of the same types of hair problems. Many women I interviewed said, "Hair problems run in my family. All the women in my family have the same hair problems." They say this to me in order to somehow validate their hair problems, and at the same time, they shift the blame away from themselves and their behavior.

At the end of the day, it is still behavior—not your age—that is the core cause. As you grew into a woman, each day somebody or something made an impression or influenced you to do certain things to your hair. As you got older, you tried new things, but you still used some of the things that you were taught as a girl, because something about it just seemed right. Well, that something is called familiarity. You use the hair methods, habits, and even products that you grew up with, which is not a problem if this familiarity is not causing aging damage to your hair and scalp.

You can control or change how your hair and scalp ages. I have found the reality for most women as they age is that their hair strands age and die away faster than they age. The changes that I would like to address are the changes that you put your hair through. We will examine the life of a single strand—the aging process of your hair strands.

Before a single strand naturally falls out of its follicle to make way for the next strand, it goes through many changes in its short life. The part of the strand that is on the surface of the scalp has three main parts: scalp hair, shaft, and end. We will examine the life of a single strand starting with the scalp hair as the hair emerges from the scalp and becomes visible. The scalp hair is the strongest part of the strand because it is the youngest part of the strand. Have you noticed that when your hair breaks, the hair close to the scalp is the last to break away? I like to call this part of the strand baby hair. It is strong because it has all of its layers, giving it the best elasticity. As the hair grows older, it pushes farther away from the scalp, obtaining length, and the body of the strand is created, called the hair shaft. The shaft of the strand is older than the scalp hair but younger than the ends. Some wear and tear is present as the shaft begins to lose elasticity, and some layers begin to lift and peel away. The last and final part of the strand is the end. The end is the oldest, which makes it the weakest part of the strand. The ends have very poor elasticity and have lost most of their protective layers because of repeated exposure to extreme wear-and-tear conditions. As your hair strand goes from young to old, and grows from scalp to end, many changes occur. The hair can go from strong to weak, but it does not have to. You may not be able to stop your hair from getting older, but you can stop the negative effects of aging hair. You can do something about it.

Just like with your body, if you take better care of your strands, you will slow the negative effects of aging. The number one thing that you must do is protect and preserve your strands. In the life of a single strand, it is exposed to many things that will affect the strand in different ways. As we care for our hair, we shampoo in order to keep the hair clean and free from debris. But this necessary step can cause aging damage in two ways. First, if you use a shampoo with a high pH, it will cause the protective layers of the shaft and end to lift, causing your strands to become dehydrated, which will cause premature aging of the strand. Second, by shampooing the hair in a rough manner and pushing the hair into the head, you can tear the shaft, causing poor elasticity of the strand, and the hair will break easily. Also, the way you handle your hair, in other words your basic grooming, is another seemingly innocent way you can expose your hair to the possibility of premature aging damage to the entire strand. Improper handling of the strands such as tugging or pulling on the hair will cause rips and tears in the shaft and on the end.

You must be careful about how you use styling tools. One styling tool that is used often—in some cases daily—is the flat or curling iron. When the shaft and end of the hair strand are overly exposed to this tool, the protective layers of the shaft simply melt away. Your hair shaft will thin, losing its fullness and taking away the youthful look of the shaft. The ends will become thin also, and split easily. Using a blow dryer causes swelling of the strands, resulting in weak spots throughout.

Finally, the most traumatic damage to the strand is caused by overexposure to chemical treatments. Applying chemical treatments to the hair improperly can cause damage to the scalp hair, shaft, and end.

Chemical damage can be fatal to your hair strand, shortening the life of the entire strand and causing you to lose your hair. All of the things that I mentioned can have a negative aging effect on your strands, and your hair will feel and look old. Aged hair will break easily, feel rough, and look dry and brittle. However, as I indicated earlier, if you have damaged your hair, you still have time to start over, but you have to be careful because you may find yourself on a roller coaster of hair problems. Remember, in each cycle of your life, from puberty to menopause, you will have a different head of the hair, but you will have the same hair problems if you continue the same bad hair care habits and don't behave properly.

As we age, our scalp also ages, because scalp is skin. The scalp sheds its top layers on a continual basis, allowing new protective layers to develop. You have an opportunity to have a youthful scalp throughout your life. Having a youthful, healthy scalp is important because it will aid in yielding youthful, healthy hair growth. Also, a healthy scalp will help resist aging scalp disorders and diseases, such as certain types of dandruff. Just as you care for the skin on your body, you must also care for your scalp.

There are seemly innocent, simple mistakes that we make in scalp care, things that we must recognize and then change in order to stop the scalp from aging. These are three of the most common areas: shampoo habits, shampoo methods, and hair products. Some women have poor shampoo habits. Many women don't shampoo their hair and scalp on a regular basis; some will wait for weeks or even months at a time between shampoos. Can you imagine not taking a bath or shower on a regular basis? I am not saying that all women need to shampoo every day, but you will need to shampoo on an as-needed basis. Remember, the scalp is shedding its dead skin cells daily, and the dry skin begins to build up after about three days. It is important to clean your scalp twice every week, or more, depending on what environment your hair and scalp are exposed to. Dust, dirt, debris, dry scalp, and hair product residue can build up, creating a home for disease-causing bacteria. This can have a negative effect on how the hair grows as well as cause aging damage to the scalp.

Other women have poor shampoo methods. Many shampoo using their fingernails or sharp shampoo brushes, scratching the scalp with sharp objects, before and during the shampoo process. Sharp objects can tear the scalp, open the scalp up to a serious scalp infection, and lead to temporary or even permanent hair loss. Poor hair products can cause problems as well. There are many products on the market with promises to give you the hair of your dreams. Some women walk around with what seems to be picture-perfect hair, but have you noticed that many of them are always scratching their scalps? Their scalps itch because most hair products address the hair style and not the care of the scalp, or the hair for that matter. Hair products are a big issue with women because we want the right one, the one that is the best to create just the right hair-style. But not all are the best for our scalp, and some will leave a filmy, negative buildup on the scalp that causes the scalp pores and the mouths of the hair follicles to become clogged, which can temporarily stop hair growth. Many products, including shampoos, conditioners, and styling lotions, leave the scalp itchy and dry. All of this causes the scalp and hair not only to look and feel old, but actually become prematurely old.

I have done scalp analyses on forty-year-old women who have scalps that looked older than those of some eighty-year-old women. I compared the skin on the face to the skin on the scalp, and the difference was unbelievable. The skin on the face was clean, smooth, shining, and hydrated. The skin on the scalp was polluted, cracked, and dry. Some will say there is a difference in scalp skin and face skin, and, yes, they are right. But the skin on your scalp and on your face have the same basic needs in order to stay youthful. All skin on the body needs to be cleaned and hydrated on a regular basis. I will speak more on the scalp as skin later in this guide.

In conclusion, it does not matter if you are going though puberty, menopause, or any age in between: your hair and scalp can look and feel young at any age. Just stop doing the negative things that age your hair and scalp, and start doing the positive things that offer youth to your hair and scalp.

Chapter Three:

How Do I Create a Foundation for Healthy Hair Growth?

Your hair is not just floating above your head; hair is an appendage of the scalp. People frequently forget that the scalp is skin. Learning about the scalp, its layers, and its connection to hair will give you a better understanding of how important it is to take care of your scalp in order to have younger-looking hair. In this chapter, you will discover the role the scalp plays in healthy hair growth at any age and the importance of remembering that the scalp is skin as it relates to anti-aging.

To realize the importance of the scalp and its life cycle, you need to understand the fact that the scalp is skin. Skin is an organ on the body whose main function is to cover the body with protective cells. Let's talk about some of the functions of the skin. One primary function is the skin's role in regulating body temperature. When we get hot, we sweat, and the purpose of sweat is to cool off our bodies. Many women comment, "I sweat more on my head than anywhere else."

This brings me to the point I want to make: The scalp is skin, and as the skin (which includes the scalp) sweats, waste and salt are flushed out and onto your body, including the skin on your head. Because our scalps have extra insulation, called hair, they may heat up more than the skin anywhere else on our bodies, which means that we will sweat more on our heads than on our torsos. That sweat and waste must be cleaned away; however, many women will shower their bodies but not shampoo their scalps and hair. Some even wait until the next salon visit or shampoo day before cleaning their hair. The type of environment that is created is negative and can cause the scalp to age as you repeatedly, month after month, keep your scalp in such a dirty situation. The aging damage will accelerate and become more apparent; your scalp will begin to itch, and as you scratch, you open the scalp up to even more serious problems.

A healthy scalp is very important to prevent scalp aging because the epidermal layers are the first line of defense, not only for their ability to hold moisture, but also for their ability to resist many dangerous chemicals in the environment as well as other things that the skin comes in contact with.

The Epidermis, Dermis, and the Hypodermis

The skin has three layers. Most of you are familiar with the epidermis and the dermis. The layer that you may not know exists is the hypodermis. I went through beauty school and part of trichology school before I even heard of the layer called the hypodermis, and it was not until I began to write my dissertation that I realized the importance of this forgotten layer. These layers are a vital part of the overall health of your body. They are of particular interest to us because the epidermis,

dermis, and hypodermis make up a fundamental part of hair growth and can influence how well your hair grows—even whether or not it grows. Unfortunately, many women and professionals act as if the hair were just floating above their heads, with little to no consideration for the scalp when styling hair. You must keep in mind that the scalp is the foundation of a healthy, youthful head of hair. Also, you must listen to the intellect that tells you hair is an appendage of the scalp, and as it is formed it flows, grows, and develops through the dermis as well as the epidermis before it becomes a solid fiber. Keeping the dermis and epidermis healthy is very important because they carry a precious cargo: the hair follicle.

The Epidermis

The epidermis is, by far, the layer that suffers the most abuse; therefore I will spend more time explaining how easily it is injured, causing aging damage. The epidermis is the outside layer of skin and is itself made up of a tier of five layers that protect the inner layers and other delicate tissues. These layers are thin and fit tightly together, shielding the body from some of the most basic airborne intruders. This protection occurs only when the epidermis is healthy, with all of its layers present.

For example, having a healthy epidermis is very important to preventing the scalp from perm burns. There are a growing number of women who experience such burning. I conducted a study to prove my theory about why women burn while having a perm, and in this study, I wanted to prove that you don't have to suffer from that reaction. I began with a questionnaire, and one question was, "Why do you think that you burn when receiving your perm?" Many women said, "I have a sensitive scalp"; some women answered, "I have always burned whenever I have gotten a chemical [service] of any type." Although I received many interesting answers, those two were the most frequent.

Here is a breakdown of the survey responses. I found that over 60 percent of the women who stated they had sensitive scalps actually had *developed* a sensitivity to chemical services after receiving perms for many months and sometimes years. My studies concluded that sensitive scalp comes from a damaged scalp. My studies also showed that the reason burning and irritation were occurring was that, over a period of time, the epidermal layers began to wear away, which is how the sensitivity developed. I proved this by creating an environment that would allow the damaged epidermis to repair itself as it grew new and healthy layers. The epidermal layers naturally peeled then shed dead skin on a continual basis as new cells develop to replace the ones that fell away. When your scalp is repeatedly exposed to unhealthy situations, it will begin to peel excessively. The peeling accelerates as the skin struggles to heal, causing a thinning out of the epidermis, which will make your scalp sensitive to chemicals. From the group of over one thousand women who were involved in this five-year study, only a small percentage, less than 5 percent, had a naturally thinner epidermis on her scalp. A worn, thin, sensitive, damaged scalp is the cause of many burns during perm applications, and this repeated damage will age the scalp, causing disorders and eventually hair loss.

A healthy epidermis is crucial to healthy hair growth, because the epidermis houses the mouth of the hair follicle, that pinhole from which the hair emerges. The epidermis also houses the mouth of oil glands that rest at the base of the mouth of the hair follicle, and the sweat glands that rest beside it. The mouth is the only part of the hair follicle that is on the outside of the skin and can be seen with the naked eye. This little opening must be cleaned on a regular basis to prevent aging damage that develops when the scalp is left in a dirty environment. On the body, dirt and dead skin cells are brushed off by our clothing or are washed away with daily showering or bathing. The process that allows the epidermal scalp to flake away dead cells is different: as the scalp goes through this same natural shedding, the hair can act as a trap, fencing the dead skin against the scalp. Couple that with the fact that many women don't shampoo on a regular basis, and you have a buildup. In addition to the dead cells that are on the scalp, there are things collected from the air and hair product residue that get into the hair, work their way to the scalp, and are trapped against the scalp. This can cause an aging effect as the scalp pores, including the mouth of the hair follicle, become clogged and polluted. As these pollutants develop, they create an environment for disease and other aging scalp disorders. I will explain in detail in a later chapter the three categories of pollutants as well as how they can cause a negative environment that causes the scalp to age.

The sebaceous, or oil, glands that rest at the base of the mouth of the hair follicle just inside the scalp are connected to the mouth of the hair follicle and will supply the scalp as well as the hair with a continual thin flow of natural oils.

Natural oils help the scalp to ward off infections, aid in healing, and are designed to lubricate both the hair and scalp. When the scalp epidermis is continually attacked and damaged through neglect, such as poor scalp care and abuse, the ability of the oil glands to aid in any way becomes compromised. Many women, particularly black women, suffer from dry scalp, and the problem accelerates when the scalp does not receive basic care. Some women will need to add oil to the scalp as part of treatment to help the skin heal. When the scalp returns to a healthy state, extra oils are no longer needed. This has been a confusing issue to some, because they have been told by their dermatologists and other hair care professionals that any oil used on the scalp will clog the pores and cause a buildup. On the contrary, it is not the oil that causes the problem. This pore-clogging problem occurs for two reasons. First, you must be sure that you are using an oil and not a heavy grease product. Second, you must be sure that your scalp does not have an existing buildup in the scalp pores.

The best way to know whether your oil is the right one and won't clog your scalp pores is to apply a small amount of the oil to the back of your hand. While rubbing it in, you should notice a slight shine to the skin, which shouldn't feel sticky to the finger. Next, rinse your hand with warm water; the oil should dissolve quickly. If the oil rinses easily, then it is safe to use and won't clog the mouth of the hair follicle or other scalp pores. Remember if the oil is skin-friendly, it will be scalp-friendly.

Some women have existing buildup of hair products, which already clogs their scalp pores. When they use an oil that normally may offer a beneficial lubricant for the scalp, the existing problems become worse; in some cases causing scalp itch. Many buildups stem from using hair and scalp care products that don't break down well in water, as well as infrequent shampooing. In severe cases of clogged pores, the scalp will need to be detoxified in order to clarify it and make the openings clean and clear. You can follow the clarifying steps I describe later in this book, which will help you clarify your scalp pores, including the mouth of the hair follicle.

The Dermis

Now let's look at the next layer, the dermis, which lies beneath the epidermis and is known as the "true" skin. Like the epidermis, the dermis has its own layers: two thick layers house the internal portion of the follicle, a tube-like impression in the scalp, as well as receptors, blood vessels, and arteries.

The Hypodermis

The hypodermis layer lies beneath the dermis. This fatty tissue works to insulate the body, conserving heat. It also contains blood vessels, lymph vessels, bases of hair follicles, and bases of the sweat glands. It connects the blood and lymph vessels to the rest of the body's systems. Hormones, nutrients, and medications are processed through the hypodermis layer. Stress also affects the hypodermis in relation to hair loss because the hypodermis layer houses the base of the hair follicle, the dermal papilla, the heart of the hair. Due to its direct connection to the body systems, the hypodermis layer actually facilitates the negative action that occurs when someone suffers from internal follicle hair loss.

As we age, our skin ages, and this aging process influences how our scalp ages. But getting older does not have to affect how healthy your scalp is. Understanding that the scalp is skin gives you a different perspective concerning your hair and scalp, allowing you to view the scalp as an important foundation for healthy hair growth. This perspective will help you realize that you have more control over the health of your scalp, and you will find that your scalp not only feels better, but also does indeed become younger. Using what you will learn as you continue through *Every Woman's Guide to Beautiful Hair at Any Age* will alert you to the damaging things that you may be doing that cause your scalp to prematurely age. And once you know what's wrong, you can start doing what's right!

CHAPTER FOUR:

HOW DOES MY HAIR GROW, AND WHY DO I LOSE IT?

In this chapter, you will learn about the hair strand, including its type and texture. You will gain a fuller knowledge of this threadlike fiber, regardless of whether you have naturally straight or curly/kinky tresses. Additionally, I will explain the role certain layers of the strand play in hair aging, which will give you a better understanding of how important it is to take care of your hair in order to have younger-looking hair. Finally, you will learn how the hair grows in cycles as this guide provides you with a better understanding of how hair ages and what the body needs in order to produce a healthy head of hair.

Hair

The hairs on your scalp are threadlike appendages made up of dead protein cells. Even though these dead fibers have no feeling, your hair can look very alive. Learning about the hair strands and understanding how they grow, whether your tresses are naturally straight or curly, will make it much easier to protect your hair from aging damage.

Hair, when in a healthy state, is pretty stable. Because hair is a dead substance, it is relatively easy to preserve the cells. In other words, with a care regimen, your hair will stay on your head for its entire life cycle. Hair has a strong resistance to damage. Your hair puts up a fight when exposed to damaging things! However, it literally will fall apart, layer by layer, before it ultimately breaks away. The hair breaks down because, even though to the naked eye, hair looks like a solid form, a single strand actually consists of three layers: cuticle, cortex, and medulla.

The outermost covering of the hair strand is called the cuticle. The cuticle consists of hard overlapping fibers that point toward the tip of your hair strand. I call the cuticle layer, the style layer; a healthy cuticle layer will determine how well your hair looks and styles. As the outside layer, the cuticle protects the interior layers and contributes to 20 percent of the overall strength of the hair.

The next layer is called the cortex; this layer contains the pigment that gives the hair its natural color. The cortex layer also is where chemical changes occur. This middle layer plays an important role in giving the hair strength and elasticity. A healthy cortex contributes about 80 percent of the overall strength of the hair.

The last of the layers, and perhaps least talked about, is the medulla, the innermost layer of the hair strand. The medulla is a hollow tube within the hair; however, the medulla is not always present in every hair strand.

Understanding Type and Texture

A large number of women are confused about two simple things as they relate to hair, and that lack of understanding is causing most of their hair dilemmas. I am talking about hair type and texture. When I asked women to tell me about their hair, I got responses such as "poker-straight hair," "good hair," "bad hair," "thick hair," "thin hair," and "coarse hair." Understanding your hair texture and type will allow you to take better care of your hair and literally may save your hair. You will be able to determine what is best for your hair—for example, how much heat your hair can tolerate and which technique of hairstyling works best with your particular hair texture and type. But first, you must have a clear understanding about each texture and type. Hair texture and type should not be described with negative phrases like, "bad hair." There is no such thing as bad hair, and as far as I am concerned, all the hair that you are blessed with is good hair!

Hair Texture

Hair texture is determined by the size of each individual hair strand. Small strands are described as thin hair, average or medium strands are described as medium hair, and large strands are described as coarse hair. Most women have multiple textures making up their hair. You may notice that your hair is coarse at the nape and fine at the crown, or the opposite may be true.

As we age, sometimes our hair texture can change, and our strands can naturally become considerably smaller than when we were younger. However, that does not mean that your hair necessarily should become noticeably thinner. What my studies have shown is that many women inflict aging damage to their hair strands, causing part or even the entire strand to thin out. When this occurs, it is called an *unnatural* texture change. A texture change occurs when the strand changes from medium to fine, from coarse to medium, or, in extreme cases, coarse to fine, as the cuticle begins to peel away layer by layer. Understanding your hair texture will help you create a personalized care program to prevent aging damage. Even if you have fine or small strands, you can still have full hair as long as your hair layers are healthy.

Aging damage causes your strands to become thinner and thinner; this is a process that will occur slowly over the life of the strand. In extreme cases of damage, the strand will lose cuticle layers to the point where there is not enough elasticity to support simply combing; subsequently, the strand breaks away before it can cycle through to the natural shedding phase. I have identified this as a hair disorder called Short Hair Syndrome (SHS). I will describe this hair disorder in length in a later chapter.

Hair Type

Hair type categorizes the shape of your strands, whether they are curly or straight. Most people have one hair type that will dominate the entire head: all curly/kinky hair or all straight hair. The important thing to remember about your hair is type (shape) is not the same as texture (size). Many get this confused, and it can lead to damage. For example, a woman with a hair type that is extremely curly/kinky may have a fine texture, but, due to the tightly coiled fiber, her hair may appear to be coarse. That mistake can lead to chemical or heat overprocessing. A small strand, despite its thick look, does not have enough support layers to withstand the same amount of heat or chemicals that coarse hair does. The analogy I give is to think of coarse hair as a tree trunk, and fine hair as a twig. Now try to imagine how many hits with an axe it will take to chop through the trunk; now imagine the twig. I think you get the picture.

Self–Strand Examination

It is very easy to learn what texture you have, as well as your type, by doing a self–strand examination. Examine your strands by sitting in front of a well-lit vanity mirror; one with some magnification would be best. Part your hair from ear to ear and down the middle of your head. Pick up the hair at the crown, and then slide a small-toothed comb through the scalp hair, resting the comb against the scalp. Next, lift the comb through the hair about two inches from the scalp through the hair and stop. Using your forefinger and thumb, hold onto the section of hair and remove the comb. Now gently, but still with a firm grip, pull your hair straight. Use your other hand to spread apart the hair that is closest to the scalp. Lean toward the mirror, and you will see clearly the size of your strands. If you slide your fingers down toward the ends, you will see how your hair may change in texture as the strand grows away from the scalp. If the hair at the scalp is thicker than the hair on the shaft and toward the ends, then you have a texture change. This self-examination will also allow your to view your natural texture.

Changes in Hair Texture and Type

Your hair may change in texture naturally as you age, but you want to be careful to prevent an unnatural texture change as your strands age through wear and tear and damage. Protect your strands so that you can preserve the texture throughout the life of each of your strands. The type of hair that you had as a child may change as you age. If you had straight hair, your hair will not become straighter; however, if you had curly hair as a child, you may find that now your hair is growing in straighter. While this is rare, such drastic type change is possible. It does not matter what texture or type of hair you have; what is important is that you have a clear understanding of the difference between the two types and the difference between the three textures, and that you know how to categorize your hair. This knowledge will help you protect and preserve your strands.

Hair Growth Cycle

Many researchers have conducted studies and have come up with various numbers and averages with regard to hair, its growth, and its growth cycle. Reviewing these professionals, I have found that their conclusions have a large range. Many of them agree that the human head has anywhere from eighty thousand to one hundred fifty thousand hair follicles. They agree also that the hair in those follicles will grow for two to six years, at a rate of one-half inch every four to eight weeks, and those same follicles are shedding eighty to one hundred fifty strands each day. Although scientists and researchers have various theories about hair growth, I have found that they all concur that hair growth occurs in phases. Each phase involves an important step, and each phase needs to be completed in order to advance to the next phase, when the time comes, so as to prevent breaking the cycle of hair growth.

Your hair grows in a three-phase cycle. The first phase is a time for your hair to grow freely for an average of two to six years. Remember ladies, for those of you who say they hate their new growth: no new growth, no hair growth! Let's say you have one hundred fifty thousand follicles, and each one grows for six years. The challenge for many women is to keep their hair for as many years as possible; in other words, to keep their hair on their heads through their full growth cycles. Properly care for your hair, and your hair will grow long and full. This sounds simple, but it is the only way that you can get the maximum length for your hair. Many women say their hair just won't grow; however, my studies have shown that the hair is growing, but parts of the individual hair shafts and ends become damaged, breaking off before any length is obtained.

After the growth cycle ends, the strand simply falls off the head through shedding. This should clear away any lingering thoughts about the possibility that the damage done to your hair as a child or teenager somehow damaged your strands for life. The hair that you had when you were younger is not the same hair that is on your head today; sweetie, that hair has been gone for years! The mere fact that your hair grows, then sheds to make room for new strands is indeed a blessing, considering the torturing and fatal damage that you put your hair through. You wouldn't have a hair on your head if you did not get all these chances for a new strand to come in and replace the old one! You have many opportunities to have youthful hair that is full and radiant. However, I must emphasize this warning: You can cause damage that not only ages your hair and shortens the life of particular strands, but also inflicts aging damage to your scalp that can cause permanent hair loss.

To understand what I am saying, we need to look a little deeper at the life of a single strand to help you understand how the hair ages. A single follicle can produce many strands during your lifetime, but not all at one time.

Anagen Phase

The most active phase is called the growth, or anagen, phase. The anagen is the longest of all the phases in the complete growth cycle. Not all of your hair strands are growing at the same time; roughly 80 to 90 percent of your hair follicles are in the anagen phase at any one time. The exact number of years the hair will grow varies between individuals; in most cases, it depends on genes. Some will have hair strands that live for two to four years; some will have strands that last for four to six years. This explains why some women can grow hair down to their backs or beyond, and some can grow hair only just below their shoulders. In rare cases, you will see women with hair like Crystal Gayle, the singer who has hair that just naturally grows to her ankles. Again, that type of hair growth is rare and strongly genetically linked. If you are trying to grow hair to your waist and beyond, it just may not be possible for you. But let's talk about what can be a natural, healthy length for you.

Your hair naturally grows at a rate of about one half-inch every four to eight weeks, which means each year your hair's length should increase somewhere between 3 to 6 inches. With the average life of a strand being four to six years, your potential hair length should be, on average, at least 12 inches and at most 36 inches. I've heard some women complain that they can't seem to obtain even 12 inches of hair in a lifetime. The reason for this lack of length is that the hair strand is falling apart and then breaking away before it can obtain its full growth potential. In a later chapter, I will share with you my own research that explains this phenomenon.

Catagen Phase

After your hair has been in the anagen phase, it lays in a dormant until it enters the next cycle, the catagen phase. The catagen is the shortest phase in your hair growth cycle, lasting only one to three weeks. However, just because your hair is not growing does not mean the hair follicle is totally inactive. The follicle is busy detaching parts of itself from its base as the dermal papilla condenses; only the cells above become inactive. The dermal papilla is the heart of the hair, the only part of your hair that has a "real life" connection to the rest of your body; it is your hair's lifeline. Lack of dermal papilla cell stimulation is the cause of growth stoppage.

Telogen Phase

Now the hair follicle enters the last phase, which is somewhat similar to the catagen phase. This stage is called the telogen phase, which lasts roughly one hundred days, and the follicle is in a resting state. In the telogen phase, the dermal papilla can become isolated in the dermis as the remaining hair follicle regresses and sits in the dermis skin. Although a follicle is resting, it may still have a hair fiber in it. When follicles enter the telogen phase and stop making hair, they dump their remaining cells onto the end of the fiber. This lump of cells acts as an anchor to hold the hair fiber in the tube of the follicle. The hair is now called club hair because the lump of cells on the end gives it a club-like appearance. This club-like tissue is better known as the hair bulb and you can see it on the end of your strand after it has fallen out.

Hair Shedding—Natural Hair Loss

A new anagen phase begins, and the growth process starts over as the hair follicle produces a new hair. As the growth within your hair follicle begins, your new hair strand that is in the mouth of the resting follicle eventually will push out the old hair, in a process called hair shedding. Many of you have heard, perhaps from your stylist, that your hair naturally sheds daily. That's true; this hair shedding process eventually happens and is how you will, at some point, lose, then regrow each of your strands in a natural way, but not all at one time. Allow me to explain further.

In the scalp of a healthy adult, approximately 90 percent of the hair will be in the anagen phase, and approximately 10 percent will be in the telogen phase. Remember, this phase lasts one hundred days, and you must also take into account that the scalp contains one hundred thousand to one hundred fifty thousand hairs, with ten thousand to fifteen thousand in the telogen phase, which makes up your 10 percent, and each day, of that 10 percent, at least 1 percent of those hairs in the telogen phase will be at the end of the one-hundred-day-long phase. This means, under normal circumstances, you can shed up to one hundred fifty strands each day. Even though this may seem like a lot of hair to lose in one day, this is a natural process and will vary at any age.

So do not be alarmed when you see some strands in your comb. Many women come into my clinic concerned about hair loss; they think their hair is shedding too much. I assure them that hair is shedding continually. This is normal, and the hair is renewed by the rotating series of growth, rest, and shedding, then the follicles renew themselves and growth starts again. Hair growth is coordinated so that each hair passes through the three phases independently. This coordination allows the total amount of hairs on the head to remain constant.

Density

Density, which is genetically linked, deals with the number of strands per square inch on your scalp. Normal density can range from slight to substantial, varying from person to person. Some individuals have hair so dense that it grows in follicle units, giving the appearance—even when viewed under a microscope—that two or more strands are growing from one follicle. Actually the two follicles are positioned extremely close together. It is important to notice when you may be experiencing a density change. A density change is when the hair per square inch begins to decrease in number.

Density Check

Checking your density is very simple; all you need is a rattail comb and a large mirror with a light above it. Lay the comb flat against the top of your forehead. Using the tail of the comb, starting at the middle of your forehead, slide the tail back toward the center of your head. Carefully lift the comb straight up and away from your head. Using your other hand, hold hair open and untangle any hairs that seem to pull. Allow your hair to fall, forming a part with some hair on the right of your head and some on the left. Pin the hair down using bobby pins to hold it in place. Look at your part. It should look even; you may have a narrow or slightly wider part, but it definitely should be even. This means that you have normal density. If the part starts narrow and then becomes wider as you look toward the crown, you have density inconsistencies in that area. In some cases, you may notice a narrow part and a circle as you look toward the crown. One last sign of a density change is if your part looks like a Christmas tree.

Density Changes

Density changes in your hair mean that the hair per square inch is not consistent, which may mean that you are in some stage of alopecia (balding). If this is the case, you need to see a trichologist for a density check. You will want one who uses a handheld microscope; this will allow the trichologist to view the mouths of the hair follicles magnified enough to be counted. During your visit, the trichologist will let you know whether this is on a surface level or not. If your trichologist has determined that the hair loss or thinning is not stemming from the surface, in other words, the epidermis and the mouth of the follicle are healthy, then the trichologist will assist you in making a decision about finding a dermatologist or other practitioner, if needed. In addition to consulting with a dermatologist, it is important to understand as much as you can about hair loss. For research, the Internet is loaded with information on this topic, but be careful about the source. Be sure that the information is coming from a reputable trichologist, dermatologist, researcher, scientist, or doctor. You will need to know the common types and the general information about each type of hair loss. Also, you can learn about what to expect during your visits to the professionals.

Strand Reading

It is important to learn how to read your hair strands, because this skill will point you in the right direction to receive the help that you need to treat your hair loss problems. Although learning to read your strands will not offer a diagnosis, it is a strong tool for alerting yourself that there is a problem that needs the attention of a specialist to determine what is causing your hair loss. Also helpful is that you will have a better idea of the type of professional needed.

As you have just learned, your hair sheds on a daily basis, and that shedding is a natural part of the hair growth process. Many women—and I suspect that includes some of you who are reading this book—are experiencing hair loss and are losing more than is natural. In my clinic, we assist individuals in learning how to read their hair strands. Many women have brought bags of hair to my clinic with one question: "Am

I supposed to lose this much hair and is this normal?" As I look at the bags of hair, the short answer is no. Allow me to elaborate. You must understand that when you think of natural shedding, it is just that: normal and unnoticeable. Remember that you are supposed to shed a maximum of one hundred fifty strands a day, and that is not very many strands considering the amount of hair on your head. Strands just fall away at random times, like when shampooing or combing your hair, or in the wind. When you find yourself at the point where you are noticing more and more hair in your comb, on your pillow, and even on your floor, then you may be experiencing multiple types of hair loss or some form of breakage. Below are some easy steps for reading your strands at home.

How to Read Your Strands at Home
1. Collect three days of strands and save them in a closeable plastic baggie.
2. Be sure to have plenty of bright light, and sit comfortably at a table.
3. Lay strands on dark paper if your hair is light in color; lay strands on light paper if your hair is dark in color.
4. Separate strands into three groups on your paper. Group one will be all the strands that have a small club-like tissue on one end; group two will be all the strands that are the length of your hair but are very thin; group three will be shorter hair strands.

If you have more strands from group one, then you are most likely shedding normally; you may want to see a trichologist just to be sure. The club-like tissue on the end is called the hair bulb. The hair bulb is the part of the strand that was once attached to the dermal papilla, the heart of the hair. The bulb is the last part of the hair strand to leave the follicle during the shedding phase. If excessive bulbs are in your baggie, you will need to have your trichologist recommend a dermatologist and possibly other medical doctors. If you have more strands from group two, you should seek the aid of a trichologist because your hair is experiencing a form of breakage called layer peeling. Also, if you have more strands from group three, you need to seek the aid of a trichologist, because your hair is experiencing a form of breakage caused by strand dehydration.

What to Expect and Where to Start

After home examinations of both your density and strands, discuss your findings with your stylist. She will be able to do a more intense and thorough density check, because she can stand over your head for a better view and make many section parts in order to check the density of your entire scalp. Also, your stylist can assist you with a strand reading if you need help. However, your stylist is not a trichologist.

The Best Approach Available

There are three approaches in treating hair loss: over-the-counter (OTC) or generic medicine, natural medicine, and pharmaceutical medicine. Some OTC products may do very little to solve your hair loss issues even though they claim to have a cure, so be careful and research the products as well as their companies. Many experts of natural and pharmaceutical medicines have various approaches to the treatment of hair loss. I encourage you to research these products and educate yourself on all the treatment options that are available to you. The three groups of experts who I have found helpful for diagnosis are trichologists, dermatologists, and endocrinologists.

Trichologists

Although trichologists have been around since the early 1900s, many of you, probably, have never heard of them. A trichologist, simply stated, is a professional who studies hair strands, their diseases and disorders, and their connection to the scalp. Similar to other practitioners, trichologists' areas of specialty may vary from one to another. Ask for a phone appointment to speak directly to the trichologist or the assistant, so that you can ask questions about your problems and get answers that will help you determine whether or not you should make an in-person appointment. I recommend that you see a trichologist who will examine your scalp and strands using a handheld microscope. A microscope that has a cable attached to a monitor would be best. This will allow you to view the examination of your scalp and strands. Keep in mind that not all trichologists use this type of equipment, so ask before making your appointment. Your visit to the trichologist is important, because you can find out if the hair loss is stemming from external issues. Be sure to ask the trichologist about the treatment options that are available from the office. Also, you should be aware that trichologists are drugless practitioners, so they will have a natural approach to any treatment. Be sure to ask what percentage of regrowth you can expect; this will keep you from becoming disappointed. In some cases dealing with aging damage to your scalp, your hair loss may be permanent, in which case a trichologist may be able to help stop future hair loss. Also, a trichologist may be able to recommend a stylist specializing in prevention of some types of hair loss. Trichologists can be valuable aids because of their focus and point of view, and the fact that they study the strand and its connection to the scalp. Also beneficial is the fact that they offer in-clinic visits and treatments. They can explain to you what to expect when dealing with a doctor or other specialist and give their opinions on which, if needed, should be involved.

Dermatologists

A dermatologist is a medical doctor who diagnoses and treats diseases and disorders of the skin, and also deals with the appendages of the skin, which includes hair. (Remember, scalp is skin!) A dermatologist possibly can treat hair loss problems that stem from internal follicle issues. Additionally, they can do a biopsy on your hair follicles in the areas where the density changes are occurring, which is something you definitely want done. Some women have had follicle biopsies and were disappointed, not because of the doctor's finding, but due to the pain during and the scarring afterward, causing a greater change in density. However, many dermatologists have special equipment to choose from for scalp follicle biopsies—one that is so small it can punch out one follicle at a time and is virtually painless. The dermatologist sends the follicle to a pathologist, who will report any findings to your dermatologist, who, in turn, will explain the pathologist's findings to you. So there is no need to be afraid of an examination that will aid in finding out whether your follicles are functioning properly. The thing to remember is to stay assertive with your dermatologist by asking questions about what is being used and what you can expect during and after the examination.

Do not stop if you have not solved your hair loss issues through visits to a trichologist or dermatologist; just stay focused and motivated to get to the bottom of your problems. A trichologist can diagnose and treat hair loss on the strand and surface levels. This means that a trichologist will be able to treat aging damage that is causing thinning or breakage of the hair strand and can treat aging damage on the mouths of the hair follicles that is causing hair loss or balding. A dermatologist can diagnose and treat scalp disorders and perform tests that may help determine the condition of the internal follicle area. Dermatologists also prescribe medication as necessary to treat scalp disorders. But you may need still other experts in the area of hair loss, particularly in cases where internal follicle hair loss is the diagnosis.

My research has led me to explore the practices of doctors in various fields of medicine. I looked at what they have to offer to women, particularly as they age and suffer from internal follicle hair loss. Most of what I found states that the treatment of all types of alopecia, including internal follicle hair loss, should fall under one certain specialty.

Endocrinologists

Because hair is a part of the skin, dermatologists were once thought to be the only practitioners who should treat it. Yet what is thought to be the cause of the most common form of internal hair loss, androgenic alopecia, is the actions of hormones, which are the focus of a different specialty—endocrinology. Therefore, the next doctor who should be on your list is an endocrinologist specializing in female hormone problems. Their areas of clinical focus include polycystic ovary syndrome (PCOS) and persistent acne, as well as increased hair growth and alopecia (scalp-hair loss). Surprisingly, few endocrinologists are trained to diagnose or treat hair loss in women. This is unfortunate because bridging the gap between specialties has made it possible to apply new knowledge about hormones to understanding and treating androgenic alopecia. The key to your success in finding the right expert is to look at experience, reputation, education, and success stories. All doctors must be trained and qualified to understand your type of hair loss. Also, ask for counseling; for all individuals who call my clinic, my consultants will offer counseling. In many cases, I will even require that I counsel some individuals before an examination. I do this as a part of a community outreach education program. I also use this as a time to answer all questions that clients may have about hair loss in general. The important thing to remember is to not give up until you are satisfied that you have explored all your options. Be careful, because just as with many other health areas, and with the fact that hair loss among women is now reaching epidemic levels, treatment for hair loss has become a big money-making business.

What Your Body Needs to Produce a Healthy Head of Hair

For most of my life, I have been in the hair field in some form or another, and it has always been my strong desire to educate. I have found that a large percentage of aging hair and scalp problems come from damage to the epidermal scalp areas as well as from the layers of the strand. I learned, while exploring all the reasons for hair loss, that nutrition plays a role. In the books, articles, and even lectures that I have written or been involved in, you may have noticed that I had very little to say about nutrition and its relationship to hair growth and loss. The reason I avoided mentioning such a connection is because I found that the mere mention of nutrition will cause many women to go on a so-called "health kick," taking a bottle of anything that says that it can stimulate hair growth. The number one danger is, if you are not careful (and many women aren't) and take too much of certain supplements, the nutrients that are supposed to help become toxic to your system. Also, I found that many women wasted a lot of money and got a lot of frustration. Even though those are good reasons for me to avoid emphasizing the nutrition connection, at some point I have to acknowledge that the overall health of your body can determine the overall health of your hair and its growth. I also have to recognize the fact that many women, particularly as they age, are malnourished and suffer from vitamin deficiencies. So, one of the first things that I ask when I notice that the surface-level hair and scalp appear unhealthy is, "Have you had a physical examination or blood work done to check the condition of your health, as well as to check other areas of nutrition?

The point I am making is that, along with the external factors, you will have to consider the internal factors. If you feel that your hair is not growing to its maximum potential or that you are losing hair, improper nutrition could be playing a role.

Proper Nutrition

To achieve and maintain proper nutrition, supplements can help. The health of your hair is in many ways directly related to how you take care of it; it's not just what you put on your hair that matters, but also what you put into your body. Healthy hair is indirectly associated with diet and nutrition. Remember, your hair is a part of your body, and just like every other part, your hair needs the correct nutrients in the precise amounts, not only to look, but to truly be its best. The proper supplements can aid in providing your body with what your system needs to grow healthy, youthful hair. You need to protect and preserve your hair after your scalp has produced this new, strong hair in order to keep the locks. How well you protect and preserve it will determine how radiant and youthful your hair looks throughout its life cycle. A supplement of protein can perform a vital role in hair growth because hair is largely comprised of protein; supplements of other vitamins, minerals, and amino acids also can help to provide what the body needs to grow healthy hair.

There are tons of hair vitamins on the market. You can find many vitamins in stores that claim to be cure-alls. So, it is important that, before taking any supplements, you consult your medical doctor or a natural medicine doctor, especially if you are on other medications.

Some medications may not work well with certain supplements, causing an allergic reaction or other dangerous side effect, and you can become very ill. This is especially important if you have impaired physical conditions. I also recommend that you seek the assistance of a supplement specialist; many health food stores have experts on staff. But note, speaking with the health store expert should be in addition to and not in lieu of speaking with your personal doctor!

There are many vitamins found in the food we eat, so maintaining a proper diet is relatively easy. You can use supplements as needed, because, if used correctly under a doctor's supervision, they will offer an advantage by improving your health, which will then benefit your hair and scalp. Some food sources improve blood circulation to the scalp, which is important for many reasons—number one being that the follicle is a tiny organ with veins and arteries that must have good circulation in order to perform properly. I have compiled a list of some vitamins that you can get from the food you eat. I have included some of the daily recommendations as well as some of the warnings that you must be aware of. Keep in mind, you should not expect overnight results; you must allow anywhere from three to six months and, in some cases, longer if there was a deficiency in your diet or your body absorption levels. Be sure to consult a nutritional expert, a dietitian, or your doctor, as well as seek the help of a supplement expert. I treat women who are in search of the one cure-all diet, and they are not happy when they discover that one does not exist. It is very important that you be persistent and consistent in whatever regimen you start.

Vitamins from the foods you eat

Vitamin A is an antioxidant that will help produce healthy sebum in the scalp. You will find vitamin A in foods such as fish liver oil, meat, milk, cheese, eggs, spinach, broccoli, cabbage, carrots, apricots, and peaches. Daily dose: 5,000 IU. Warning: More than 25,000 IU daily is toxic and can have an adverse consequence, causing hair loss and other serious health problems.

Vitamin C is an antioxidant that helps maintain the health of the skin and hair. You will find vitamin C in foods such as citrus fruits, strawberries, kiwi, cantaloupe, pineapple, tomatoes, green peppers, potatoes, and dark green vegetables. Daily dose: 60 mg.

Vitamin E is an antioxidant that enhances scalp circulation. You will find vitamin E in foods such as cold-pressed vegetable oils, wheat germ oil, soybeans, raw seeds and nuts, dried beans, and leafy green vegetables. Daily dose: up to 400 IU. Warnings: Can raise blood pressure and reduce blood clotting. People taking high-blood-pressure medication or anticoagulants should check with their doctors before taking vitamin E supplements.

Biotin helps produce keratin, which is the protein that the hair is mostly composed of; some studies have shown that biotin may prevent graying and hair loss. You will find biotin in foods such as brewer's yeast, whole grains, egg yolks, liver, rice, and milk. Daily dose: 150 to 300 mcg.

Inositol has been shown to keep hair follicles healthy at the cellular level. You will find inositol in foods such as whole grains, brewer's yeast, liver, and citrus fruits. Daily dose: up to 600 mg.

Niacin (vitamin B3) is known to promote scalp circulation. You will find vitamin B3 in foods such as brewer's yeast, wheat germ, fish, chicken, turkey, and other meats. Daily dose: 15 mg. Warning: Taking more than 25 mg a day can result in niacin flush—a temporary heat sensation due to blood cell dilation.

Pantothenic acid (vitamin B5) has shown in some studies to prevent graying and some forms of hair loss. You will find vitamin B5 in foods such as whole grain cereals, brewer's yeast, organ meats, and egg yolks. Daily dose: 4 to 7 mg.

Vitamin B6 has been shown to prevent some forms of hair loss. It also helps create melanin, which gives hair its color. You will find vitamin B6 in foods such as brewer's yeast, liver, whole grain cereals, vegetables, organ meats, and egg yolks. Daily dose: 1.6 mg. Warning: High doses can cause numbness in hands and feet.

Vitamin B12 aids in the prevention of hair loss. You will find vitamin B12 in foods such as chicken, fish, eggs, and milk. Daily dose: 2 mg.

Calcium is essential for healthy hair growth. You will find calcium in foods such as dairy, tofu, fish, nuts, brewer's yeast, beans, lentils, and sesame seeds. Daily dose: up to 1,500 mg. Warnings: Too much calcium can inhibit the absorption of zinc and iron. Some studies have shown that an acid found in chocolate can inhibit calcium absorption.

Chromium helps prevent hyperglycemia and hypoglycemia, both of which can cause some forms of hair loss. You will find chromium in foods such as brewer's yeast, liver, beef, and whole wheat bread. Daily dose: up to 120 mg. Warning: If you are allergic to yeast, you should not take chromium supplements.

Copper helps prevent some forms of hair loss as well as defects in hair color and structure. You will find copper in foods such as shellfish, liver, green vegetables, whole grains, eggs, chicken, and beans. Daily dose: up to 3 mg. Warning: Some studies have shown that high levels of copper can have an adverse effect and may lead to dry hair, hair loss, and severe health problems.

Iodine helps regulate thyroid hormones and has been known to prevent dry hair and some forms of hair loss. You will find iodine in foods such as fish, seaweed, kelp, iodized salt, and garlic. Daily dose: 150 mcg.

Iron prevents anemia and some forms of hair loss. You will find iron in foods such as liver, eggs, fish, chicken, whole grains, green vegetables, and dried fruits. Daily dose: 15 mg. Warning: Too much iron can lead to malfunctions of the liver and spleen.

Magnesium works with calcium to promote healthy hair growth. You will find magnesium in foods such as green vegetables, wheat germ, whole grains, nuts, soybeans, chickpeas, and fish. Daily dose: 280 mg.

Manganese has been helpful in preventing slow hair growth, aiding hair to grow closer to its normal rate. You will find manganese in foods such as whole grain cereals, eggs, avocados, nuts, seeds, beans, peas, fish, chicken and other meats. Daily dose: 3 to 9 mg.

Potassium helps to regulate blood circulation and promotes healthy hair growth. You will find potassium in foods such as avocados, bananas, lima beans, brown rice, dates, figs, dried fruit, garlic, nuts, potatoes, raisins, yams, and yogurt. Daily dose: 3,500 mg.

Selenium aids in promoting a healthy scalp, and keeping the skin and scalp supple and elastic. You will find selenium in foods such as brewer's yeast, fish, grains, tuna, and broccoli. Daily dose: 55 mcg. Warning: An excess of selenium can be toxic, causing an adverse effect leading to hair loss as well as loss of nails and teeth.

Silica strengthens hair and prevents some types of hair loss. You will find silica in foods such as seafood, rice, soybeans, and green vegetables. Daily dose: 55 mcg. Warning: An excess of silica can be toxic, causing an adverse effect, leading to the loss of hair, nails, and teeth.

Sulfur (methyl-sulfonyl-methane or MSM) is one of the main components to hair's structure. You will find sulfur in foods such as onions, garlic, eggs, asparagus, meat, fish, and dairy products. Daily dose: 1 to 3 g.

Zinc and vitamin A work together; a deficiency in either can lead to dry hair and oily skin. You will find zinc in foods such as spinach, sunflower seeds, mushrooms, whole grains, red meat, and brewer's yeast. Daily dose: 12 mg. Warning: Too much zinc can interfere with iron absorption.

Remember to consult your doctor before taking any supplements.

CHAPTER FIVE:

HOW DO MY SCALP AND STRANDS BECOME DEHYDRATED?

Your scalp can dehydrate and age just like the skin on your face, because, as I have been reminding you, scalp is skin. And guess what? Your hair can dehydrate as well. In this chapter, you will learn what you may be doing to cause scalp dehydration and hair disaster. Also, you will learn how and what you can do to prevent premature aging of your scalp and hair strands.

We often hear about how the skin on our face and other body parts can become dehydrated, but you seldom hear about how your hair and scalp can dehydrate. The fact is that many women are suffering from extremely dehydrated scalps and hair, which causes aging damage that leads both to scalp disorders and loss of hair. Hair and scalp dehydration is mostly self-inflicted. Many women believe that scalp and hair dehydration comes from not drinking enough water, but that isn't true. You can drink gallons of the purest water each and every day, and you will not prevent scalp nor hair dehydration. Although water will hydrate the inner body, it will provide very little hydration to the epidermal scalp and nothing to the hair. This is important to remember, because having hydrated scalp and hair strands is a fundamental part of the anti-aging process.

Scalp Dehydration

When something is applied to the hair, whether it is a chemical or any other hair product, it has an effect on the scalp and epidermis, sometimes causing aging damage. Cleansing, conditioning, and styling products commonly are used and are important in the care and grooming of your hair. One of the most common, seemingly harmless products that everyone uses on a regular basis is a shampoo, but some shampoos can cause negative aging damage to your scalp. Nowadays, there are many kinds of shampoo on the market. There are shampoos that claim to moisturize and condition the scalp, some even claim to stop scalp itch and flakes, and the list of promises goes on. Take, for example, dandruff shampoos: These shampoos have ingredients that are antifungal and antibacterial, and they are designed to stop scalp flaking and itch. The problem with some of these OTC shampoos, as well as prescription shampoos, is that in some cases, their ingredients will leave the scalp dehydrated. The drying effect these shampoos have on the scalp will result in scalp peeling. So, in many cases, you are defeating the purpose of using them! A dehydrated scalp will itch and flake, and those are the two main complaints that I hear from women regarding their scalps. Also, as the problem progresses, the scalp will feel tight and tender to the touch.

On the other hand, a healthy epidermis has the ability to hold the amount of moisture needed to hydrate the scalp, and the scalp's oil glands will provide a natural lubrication that will seal in that natural moisture. The scalp is exposed to a tremendous number of factors that will prohibit this natural moisturizing process from occurring, thereby depleting the scalp's moisture and causing a drop in the moisture levels of the scalp. You may be wondering how this is possible.

The epidermis, as I explained earlier, is made up of layers, and these layers protect the inner layers and other cells and tissues. When the epidermal layer becomes damaged or injured, the body goes on the defense as it works frantically to shed the damaged epidermal scalp. In many cases, when the epidermis is damaged, the dermis becomes exposed, and a sore may develop. As the epidermal scalp goes though the healing and recovering process, the sore may become runny and ooze yellow pus. The presence of this pus is actually important because it is full of your body's natural antibodies, which are designed to aid in the healing of the skin. Next, the scalp grows a scab over the exposed dermal area as it tries to heal underneath and within. As the scalp struggles to heal, you may notice it becomes tender. Additionally, in the final stages of healing, you may experience an itch and a tightness of the scalp as it literally cracks open, causing the protective scab to peel, causing a flaky dandruff. Because the epidermal layers hold moisture, when they shed excessively, their loss leaves the scalp dry. Scalp dehydration is the negative aftereffects of scalp damage.

There are several common causes of scalp dehydration, some as simple as using a high-pH shampoo. A secretion from the scalp called acid mantel is formed from the sweat glands. Oil glands give the scalp its pH, which is somewhere between 4.5 and 5.5. This pH level makes the scalp and hair acidic in reaction. In other words, the scalp and hair naturally respond in a positive way. (A pH level of 7 is neutral; anything higher is a base, which responds negatively in reactions.) All parts of the body are healthier when the basic chemistry is not disturbed, so it is very important to use a shampoo that is mildly acidic to protect the scalp. To understand this better, let's take a look at the pH scale, which allows you to read whether a liquid substance is alkaline (base) or acid. The values on the scale are from 0 to 14, with neutral being 7.

For years, women were told that they needed to balance their scalps

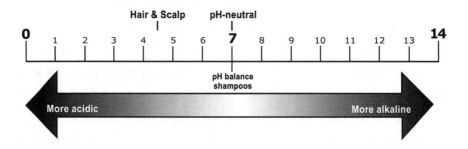

and hair by using a pH-balanced shampoo (e.g., a shampoo with a pH of 7). For a period of time, there were a number of ads that recommended buying a pH-balanced shampoo, but, strangely, you don't hear those ads anymore. The reason that you don't hear them is, studies have shown that the scalp and the hair closest to the scalp have a pH of 4.5 to 5.5, which is one hundred times more acidic than the neutral pH of 7.

So, as many women used these highly advertised pH-balanced shampoos, their scalps became dry, itchy, and even flaky. Even the scalps of women with oily scalps eventually became dehydrated. Worse, women with naturally dry scalps experienced extreme dehydration. In some cases, this occurred after just one use. You can build a better foundation for a healthy hair and scalp if you start with a shampoo that offers some anti-aging results. Shampoo is a product that we all should use on a regular basis, no matter what type of hair we have. By using a shampoo that is acid-balanced and not pH-balanced, you will clean your scalp without disturbing the basic chemistry of the hair and scalp. As a result, the scalp and hair have a better chance to prevent one of the most common causes of scalp dehydration.

At the stage when dehydration develops, the scalp will begin to age prematurely as it goes into a stage of damaging extreme dehydration. Some symptoms are itchiness, tenderness, flakes, and redness as the scalp struggles to respond, trying to heal. Many women alleviate the itchy symptom by scratching, and when they are not scratching, they are rubbing. All of this only makes the problem worse! Although it will offer some immediate relief from your itch, scratching the scalp actually increases the speed and amount of damage, because the more you scratch, the more your scalp itches, which will make you want to scratch even more. When you make a habit of scratching your scalp, you could be creating what may start out as microscopic tears on the scalp area, and the epidermal scalp will begin to wear away, becoming tender and sore, as nerve endings and receptors that lay within respond.

Women will use whatever object is in their hands—pens, combs, fingernails—and just scratch away. I have even noticed TV talk show hosts scratch, and I'm shocked, even though scratching seems like a natural thing to do. But it is in no way a natural thing to do! As a part of a study that I conducted called "Scalp as Skin," I was able to prove that persistent scalp scratching eventually will lead to aging damage and hair loss. As I counseled individuals about the dangers of scalp scratching and warned against doing this, I found that many would react by rubbing instead. However, this solution isn't much better, because while rubbing won't create tears like scratching, it does bruise the scalp. Continual rubbing causes the epidermis to become worn and thin, causing moisture loss and causing the scalp to become more sensitive and susceptible to tears and aging damage. Your scalp should never be exposed to continual rubbing unless it is completely hydrated, in other words, during shampooing. It is safe to rub your scalp during shampooing, because the hydrated scalp allows your fingers to glide across it while massaging.

If your scalp is itchy, remember that it is only an indication of some underlying problem. An itchy scalp is like a headache: It is telling you something is wrong, and you need to take action. A scalp itch may mean a number of things; to name a few, it may mean that your scalp is involved in the recovery process after damage, or it is dehydrated, or something as simple as its being dirty. If you suffer with a persistent scalp itch, don't ignore it; it may lead to scalp infections, which could lead to hair loss. Here is a little tip: If you find yourself in a situation where a sudden itch occurs, don't scratch or rub. Instead, place your forefinger and thumb under your hair, against your scalp. Simply apply pressure to the area. If the itch seems deep, then move just the skin of the scalp—but not your fingers—with a wiggle as you apply pressure.

This will give instant relief without the damaging side effects that are associated with scratching.

Try to notice every signal that your scalp is sending, and don't ignore the warning signs, because all of them stem from something. Instead of responding to an itch by scratching or rubbing, start with simply cleaning your scalp. Also, oil your scalp while it is wet, right before you dry and style your hair. If you find yourself suffering from serious chronic scalp problems, then consult a dermatologist. Most importantly, I agree with the theory that an ounce of prevention is worth a pound of cure. So take care of your scalp by protecting it with a clean, slightly acidic, stimulated, and hydrated environment. Clean your scalp by shampooing regularly, at least twice a week, using an acid-balanced shampoo. Stimulate your scalp while it is hydrated, using deep tissue massage. Seal in hydration with oil as needed.

Before we look at strand dehydration, its causes, and the aging damage that surrounds it, we need to understand clearly that scalp dehydration could shorten the life of your damaged strand. What you must keep in mind is that the scalp is the platform of your hair, and without that foundation, the appendage (hair) would be nonexistent.

Strand Dehydration

Yes, like your skin, your hair can become dehydrated. Hair is composed mostly of protein, which is a hard substance that must be balanced with moisture. Most researchers agree that hair is about 97 percent protein and 3 percent moisture. Three percent does not seem like a lot, but it is enough to give the layers of your strand softness, flexibility, and elasticity, thereby allowing the strand to be strong and shiny.

When we discussed the layers of the strand earlier, we talked about all three layers: the cuticle, the cortex, and the medulla. The layers that we will focus on here are the cuticle and cortex. Because the cuticle layer is positioned on the outside, it is exposed. The cuticle layer will suffer when the strand is under attack. As the strand wears away, the cortex layer is exposed, resulting in dehydration and ultimately causing aging damage. When the cortex is exposed, the hair becomes weak and depleted of its moisture. Hydration is vital in the stability of your hair, which is why, when your hair feels dry and brittle, you will notice also an increase of hair in your comb.

Luckily, it is not difficult to keep the hair hydrated. As a matter of fact, it is simple. Start by looking at your basic care regimen. Let's review how important shampoo pH is to the hair. The hair gets its pH from the scalp's acid mantel, which gives the hair strand a pH of 4.5 to 5.5. The pH of your hair rises as the hair grows farther away from the scalp. Also, the pH changes as the hair is exposed to hair products and the environment. As with your scalp, your hair will benefit greatly if cleansing products (e.g., shampoos) are in the range of the hair's natural pH, which is mildly acidic. Some women, particularly women with curly/kinky hair, have naturally dry hair, and many complain that their hair just won't hold moisture. They claim to have tried every hair lotion, oil, and moisturizer, and nothing seems to work, which causes many to wonder, "Am I drinking enough water?" Your scalp and hair will reap some benefits from your keeping your body hydrated, but drinking water will do little for the scalp and hair if the outside factors are not addressed.

When I examine the hair strands of someone who is complaining of dry hair problems, as a trichologist, naturally I am going to look at the external factors first. One of the things I try to determine is whether or not there is some type of blockage in the cuticle layer preventing the hair from receiving the benefits of a moisturizing conditioner or some other support product such as a leave-in cream moisturizer. That buildup must be removed before your hydration products can work. I have found that many women use leave-in products that are not water soluble, which results in buildup on the hair and scalp. This negative buildup actually creates a blockage that will not allow moisturizers to penetrate and provide benefits to the hair layers. In order to remove the buildup, the hair will need to be clarified and put in a pure, natural state. Once that occurs, moisturizing products will aid in raising the moisture levels, thereby hydrating the hair strands and increasing the overall strength of your hair.

There are many reasons why your hair becomes dehydrated, but most stem from the fact that your hair is suffering from poor porosity. Hair porosity is the hair's ability to absorb moisture. With good porosity, the cuticle layers and the cortical fibers are tight, which makes your hair resistant, meaning it won't lose its natural moisture and won't dry out easily. With average porosity, the cuticle is slightly raised, the hair appears normal, and the moisture levels seem stable but can become out of balance if regular moisturizing treatments are not done. With poor porosity, the cuticle is lifted, the hair is overporous and will process perms and colors quickly, and the moisture levels are always low because the cuticle layers are damaged, exposing the cortex to over-processing. Poor porosity will cause aging damage to your strands, manifesting in a dull-looking and dry-feeling aged strand. In cases of prolonged and extreme dehydration, the end result most likely will be hair loss.

Dry Environments

A healthy cuticle layer will hold moisture, but the moisture is depleted when the hair is exposed to hot, dry environments and extremely cold conditions. You don't have to travel outside your city or even outside your house in order for your hair and scalp to be exposed to an extremely dehydrating, aging, and damaging situation. There are times we place our hair and scalp in severe conditions and don't even know it.

I will tell you the two most common ways, which many think are harmless, that we dehydrate our hair. I have mentioned already the dehydrating effects that high-pH shampoos have on your hair. The next one came as a shock to me, and it was right under my nose. I have always believed that some of the styling tools used by many on a regular basis were drying out their hair, and I have conducted various studies that lead to that conclusion. However, it was amazing to learn what I found in some of my studies. I styled hair for over ten years before I entered the trichology program and became a trichologist, during which time I was always trying to find a way to dry the hair as I styled it, without drying out the strands. I eliminated all heated tools and simply refused to use the blow dryer. I even tried using so-called "protective products" to roller-set my clients' hair, but the hair still would dry out. My studies allowed me to focus on and look at ways that the hair was being dried out during styling. When styling your hair, there are two basic ways to dry your hair: blow drying and sitting under the dryer. Of the two, I believed that if I sat a client under the dryer, her hair would not dry out. But I was shocked to learn that roller setting the hair and sitting under the dryer could be dehydrating. What I discovered was that the scalp and the hair close to the scalp would dry, but the ends and middle of the strand still would be wet. This meant that the dryer time needed to be extended in order to dry the entire strand. The problem was that the scalp and the hair closest to the scalp would dry out, causing extreme dehydration. The entire scalp, especially the crown, would itch and the hair would feel dried out by the time the client got out from under the dryer. Although I had concluded that sitting under the dryer was one of the safer ways to dry your hair, the extended drying time and the extremely dry and hot conditions that the hair and scalp were exposed to were nevertheless the cause of the aging and dehydrating damage to both the hair and the scalp. Fortunately, my studies also led me to find truly safe yet simple ways to dry your hair.

How to Prevent Hair and Scalp Dehydration

- Air dry your hair as much as possible. No matter if your hair is curly or straight, drying it naturally is safe. Your hair will dry at a slow pace without chance of over-drying.
- Never preheat the hair dryer, and always keep it on medium setting.

If you sit under a hot dryer, you will begin to sweat, and your scalp will start to dry out because of the sudden and extreme temperature change. Your hair, scalp, and dryer should heat up at the same time. You may find yourself in a situation where you cannot control whether or not the dryer is already hot, for example, in a salon where the dryers are used all day and never allowed to cool down. I recommend two things. First, take a bottle of cold water with you and sip it when you are under the dryer. This will keep you cool, preventing your body from overheating. Second, place the dryer on cool for three minutes before sitting under it, and then turn it back to medium, allowing the dryer and your hair and scalp to heat up at the same time.

- Always rotate your rollers. Before the ends and middle of the strand can dry, the scalp and the hair closest to the scalp will begin to dry out. After five to fifteen minutes, have your stylist rotate your rollers in the opposite direction and continue until your hair is dry. By doing so, the ends and middle of the strand will dry as fast as the scalp hair. Some simple steps and changes can make a big difference!

- Watch your dryer time, and never allow extended time. In other words, come out from under the dryer the minute your hair is dry. Think about it: once your hair is dry, there is nothing left for it to do but to dry out.

- Hydrate your scalp hair, crown, and hair on the outside or top of each roller. These areas will dry out fastest because these areas are exposed to the greatest amount of heat. I recommend that you apply a very small amount of moisturizer to those areas the minute they dry. By rehydrating those areas, they will not dry out as you dry the other areas of the strand.

How your hair looks is important to you, but you will never have a nice looking hairstyle if your hair is dehydrated. Therefore, you should monitor heated styling tools. Find ways to dry and style your hair without drying it out, and remember that the degree of dry heat your hair and scalp are exposed to makes the difference. Hydrated hair is possible through safe styling, resulting in a nice, healthy-looking style.

Why Dry Environments Will Dry Out Your Hair

When you travel, you go through different climates. Your hair could become dehydrated if the moisture levels drop. Also, during the winter months, your hair goes through environmental changes that are traumatically dehydrating, just in the course of a single day. You may have never thought about this, but if you live in the part of the country where the air is always dry or the winters are cold and dry, your hair and scalp have had the experience that I am about to explain to you. Let's start with a cold winter morning. Most of us keep our house toasty (dry heat), we go outside (dry cold), and we get in the car and turn on the heater (dry heat). We get to work and walk from the car (dry cold) to inside the warm building (dry heat). That is five different and very drying situations that your hair just went through. My studies have shown that women complain about dry hair and scalp problems more during the winter months than at any other time of the year. There is good reason for this tendency: namely, the dehydrating changes that the scalp and hair go through.

Another environmental change that can cause your hair to become dehydrated is what I call transition weather. This is the weather we experience in the time between seasons, for example, when winter is ending and spring is just about to begin, with cold mornings and warm evenings. Your scalp and hair will become dry because of the temperature changes. Have you ever noticed how dry and ashy your hands and feet are in the winter or during weather changes? Because the air is dry, moisture is being pulled from whatever is moist, in this case, your skin, hair, and scalp. And if your hair and scalp have low moisture levels, extreme dehydration and aging damage set in. The key is to be prepared. Most of us use more lotion on our bodies during the dry months and never make the connection that what happens to our skin happens to our hair and scalp as well. They, too, will benefit from adding moisture.

Ways to Prevent Dry Weather Dehydration

I recommend that you apply a deep moisturizing conditioner an additional time during the week. Also, you should apply a small amount of moisturizer each day to your hair. By doing so, you protect your hair and prevent aging dehydration. In extreme cases and with coarse hair texture, in addition to applying moisturizer, apply oil on top to seal in the hydration that the moisturizer has provided.

CHAPTER SIX:

WHAT CAN I DO ABOUT HAIR LOSS AND THINNING?

In this chapter, you will learn about types of alopecia (baldness, hair loss), both internal and external. You will read about types of internal follicle hair loss and treatment options, as well as about external follicle hair loss and the telltale signs and causes of certain types of hair loss. I will help you understand your hair strands and hair-loss patterns. This will help you to determine which type of hair loss you might be suffering from.

Myths about Hair Loss

There are many myths about hair loss, and before we can understand the truth, we must clear up the myths. Here I have listed some of the most common ones and explain what truth, if any, there is to them.

Frequent shampooing contributes to hair loss. The truth is, it's not how often you shampoo. Remember, you should shampoo on an as-needed basis. For example, if your hair and scalp are oily or are exposed to polluted, dirty, or sweaty environments, you may find yourself having to shampoo every day. The key is to use a mildly acidic shampoo, remembering to be gentle as you massage it through your hair.

Hats and wigs cause hair loss. The truth is hats and wigs don't cause hair loss; it is the improper protection while wearing them that can cause hair loss. Wear a thin satin turban instead of a stocking cap under your wig. Also, wear loose-fitting hats and caps. A cap or hat is too tight if it rubs the hairline. Rubbing causes friction, and the irritation that occurs will result in hair loss.

One hundred strokes of the hairbrush daily will create healthier hair. The truth is, not all brushes are created equal. Bristle brushes will tear the hair and cause damage, so stay away from them. If you brush your hair and scalp with a flat paddle brush with little balls on the bristles, your scalp will receive a massage and your scalp oils will be distributed evenly from your scalp to the ends of your hair shaft. The thing to remember is that, if your hair is tangled or curly/kinky, you may pull and damage your strand—so be careful.

Permanent hair loss is caused by perms, colors, and other cosmetic treatments. The truth is, damage from chemicals and cosmetic treatments will cause permanent hair loss only if the hair follicle is fully destroyed, in other words scarring of the scalp occurs.

Shaving your head will cause your hair to grow back thicker. Yes and no. Yes, if your hair strands have been thinned out due to some type of aging damage, and you shave that hair off and end the life of that particular head of hair; you will have an opportunity to obtain new growth, which will be thicker than the strands you shaved off. No, if you shave healthy hair off; it will continue to grow with the same, normal, true texture.

Standing on your head will increase blood circulation and thereby stimulate hair growth. The truth is, your hair follicles are tiny little organs, and although good blood supply and circulation are important, I don't think standing on your head is going to do anything to promote them. Deep-tissue scalp massage is better.

Dandruff causes permanent hair loss. The truth is, dandruff, if left untreated, can lead to serious scalp problems that eventually will cause surface balding.

There are cosmetic products that cause the hair to grow thicker and faster. The truth is, there are products that make many claims, but only a miracle will increase hair growth and change texture beyond what is normal for your hair follicles. There are, however, hair and scalp products that can protect and care for your hair and scalp, as well as aid in the healing of your scalp. This will create an environment for healthy hair growth on a surface level.

Stress causes permanent hair loss. The truth is, there are some types of internal hair loss that are caused by stress, which I will talk about in later in this chapter. This type of hair loss is usually temporary.

Hair loss does not occur in the late teens or early twenties. The truth is, hair loss can occur at any age, but not all hair problems stem from the same source. I recommend that you use the knowledge that I'm sharing with you in *Every Woman's Guide to Beautiful Hair at Any Age*, then see a trichologist or visit a dermatologist. The most important thing to remember is, you are not defined by your hair, but your hair is a gift, so don't stop until you are satisfied that you have done all that you could to reverse the hair loss.

There is a cure for androgenetic alopecia. No, there is no known cure for this type of hair loss. I will explain in detail later in this chapter.

As We Age

The most common things that many women worry about as they age are hair loss and hair thinning. There are two basic categories of hair loss: internal follicle and external follicle hair loss. Internal follicle hair loss is when you are losing the entire strand, hair bulb included, and that hair loss is coming from the internal part of the hair follicle. External follicle hair loss is when you are losing part of the strand or losing it in certain areas; this type of hair loss comes from the mouth of the hair follicle or on the shaft itself.

So that you have a better understanding, I will describe the types of internal and external follicle hair loss. I feel too much mystery and too many unanswered questions surround hair loss. Many women are very confused about hair loss, thinking that hair loss means that they are sick or under too much stress. I think it is important for proper and effective hair care that you understand each category and some of their types, as well as causes and treatments. Allow me to share with you some of my ground-breaking research as I explored the two types of hair loss.

Internal Follicle Hair Loss

Studies show that hair loss affects approximately one-third of all women. Although hair loss is most commonly seen after menopause, it can begin as early as puberty. Normally, hair sheds from the follicle and falls out each day. Fortunately, these hairs are replaced. True hair loss occurs when lost hairs are not regrown or when the hair shed daily exceeds normal shedding. Studies show that, genetically, hair loss can come from either parent's side of the family. Internal follicle hair loss is premature; in other words, the entire strand falls out of the follicle while it is still in its growth stage. You will see large amounts of hair in your comb and on your pillowcase, and the strands will all have hair bulbs on them.

Diet and Dieting

Internal follicle hair loss may also occur due to dieting. Diet programs that have become popular are designed or administered under the direction of a "diet guru" with prescribed meals, dietary supplements, and vitamin ingestion. Sometimes the client is told that vitamins are a necessary part of the program to prevent hair loss associated with dieting. However, many medical doctors believe that vitamins cannot prevent hair loss associated with rapid, significant weight loss. Furthermore, many of the supplements are high in vitamin A, which can increase hair loss. Also, many individuals suffer from malnourishment when their regular diets do not supply the important vitamins and minerals needed to maintain proper health.

Physical and Emotional Stress and Hormonal Considerations

Telogen effluvium is not very common, but there are some types that occur more frequently. These are physical stress (e.g., surgery, illness, anemia, rapid weight change), emotional stress (e.g., mental illness, death of a family member), thyroid abnormalities, medications (e.g., high doses of vitamin A, blood pressure medications, gout medications), and hormonal causes (e.g., pregnancy, birth control pills, menopause).

Surgeries and severe illnesses can cause hair loss in rare cases. The body simply shuts down production of hair during these stressful periods because it is not necessary for survival. Instead, the body devotes its energies toward repairing vital structures and processes. In many cases, there is a three-month delay between the actual event and the onset of hair loss. Furthermore, there may be another three-month delay prior to the return of noticeable hair regrowth. This means that the total hair loss and regrowth cycle can last six months or possibly longer. Some health conditions that may go undetected can contribute to hair loss, for example, anemia (i.e., low blood count) and thyroid abnormalities. Both of these conditions can be detected by a simple, inexpensive blood test.

Hormonal changes are a common cause of female hair loss. Many women do not realize that their hair may thin after pregnancy or following the discontinuation of birth control pills. Remember, the hair loss may be delayed by three months following the hormonal change, and then another three months will be required for new growth to be achieved fully.

Anagen effluvium generally is due to medications taken internally. It is important to voice your concerns and ask your doctor if you can take an alternative medication, one that does not have the side effect of hair loss. Also, many chemotherapy treatments agents will cause hair loss because they are designed to kill off the cancer cells, which are dividing cells. Hair follicles are also dividing cells; therefore, while chemotherapy is doing its job to kill the cancer cells, it is also inhibiting the hair follicles from growing hair. Chemotherapy drugs are poisonous to the hair root cells that are responsible for hair shaft formation. Unfortunately, hair is usually lost rapidly in large quantities during treatment. When I examined the scalps of women who had gone through chemotherapy, I noticed how dehydrated and irritated their scalps were. I recommend a scalp program to balance the epidermal scalp. Keeping the scalp healthy during this process will help to assure that the mouth of the hair follicle is healthy and ready for the new hair that will grow. No hair growth stimulants, shampoos, conditioners, or other cosmetic treatments can prevent or retard this type of hair loss. The good news, however, is that once chemotherapy is completed, the hair usually grows back.

How and When Hair Regrowth Occurs

Adequate hair growth may take six months to one year. Returning hair may be different from the hair that was lost. Due to the absence or alteration of pigment, the hair may grow back white, gray, or a different color. Eventually, as the pigment cells return to normal, the original color should return. It is common for the new hair to be finer in texture initially, but, like color, the texture should return to its original thickness. It is sometimes difficult to be patient, but as the body is returning to normal and getting over the significant trauma, time is a necessary factor.

Female Pattern Baldness

Female pattern baldness (FPB), a form of internal hair loss in women, usually starts after menopause, when production of the female hormone estrogen slows down dramatically or stops altogether. Before menopause, when production of estrogen is high, this hormone has a protective effect against the small amount of testosterone that women also produce. The enzyme 5-alpha in scalp tissue reeducates and converts circulating free testosterone to DHT (dihydrotestosterone). The hormone DHT can harm hair follicles by making them shrink or by causing them to enter prematurely into the resting stage of the hair cycle. Before menopause, the estrogen in a woman's body counteracts the small amount of testosterone she produces and makes it less available to conversion to DHT. Not all women will develop FPB as they enter menopause, because this type of internal follicle hair loss is genetically linked.

Treatment Options

FPB is permanent. In most cases, it is mild to moderate. No treatment is required if a woman is comfortable with her appearance. The only drug or medication approved by the United States Food and Drug Administration (FDA) to treat FPB is minoxidil, used topically on the scalp. It may help hair to grow for 20 to 25 percent of the female population, and in the majority, it may slow or stop the loss of hair. More and more manufacturers of hair loss products are using minoxidil as an active ingredient with the recommended twice-daily use. For women, the 2 percent concentration of minoxidil is recommended. Hair loss recurs when minoxidil's use is stopped.

Hair replacement

Hair transplants are one option for women who have permanent hair loss. Hair transplantation consists of removing tiny plugs of hair from areas where the hair is continuing to grow and placing them in areas that are balding. This can cause minor scarring in the donor areas and carries a modest risk for skin infection. The procedure usually requires multiple transplantation sessions and may be expensive. Results, however, are often excellent and permanent. Be sure to seek a dermatologist who specializes in hair transplant surgery.

Hair weaving and hairpieces offer a change of hairstyle, may disguise hair loss, and improve cosmetic appearance. Although these are less expensive, they may not be the safest methods of replacing hair to cover FPB. Hair replacement techniques vary; sometimes the same type of replacements can be applied differently depending on the hair replacement center. It is important that you have an expert in that area who will explain the process and application, so that you can make an educated decision on whether or not this is an option you want to explore. Remember to ask complete questions and wait for complete answers.

Alopecia Areata

Alopecia areata, a form of internal follicle hair loss, is considered an autoimmune disease in which the immune system, which is designed to protect the body from foreign invaders such as viruses and bacteria, mistakenly attacks the hair follicles. This can lead to hair loss on the scalp and elsewhere. In most cases, hair falls out in small, round patches about the size of a quarter. Luckily, in many cases, the disease does not extend beyond a few bare patches. But for some people, hair loss is more extensive. Although uncommon, the disease can progress to cause total loss of hair on the head (alopecia areata totalis) or complete loss of hair on the face and body as well as the head (alopecia areata universalis).

These are only a few of the common complaints heard by physicians and other hair loss specialists on a daily basis. First, you should have a trichologist perform an examination using a handheld microscope to ensure that the hair follicle mouth is healthy. The AHLC suggests that you have your hair loss diagnosed by a competent dermatologist who sees hair loss patients on a regular basis. Once you know the diagnosis, you will have a better understanding of exactly which treatment option may be best for you.

Treatment Options

If the affected region is small, it may be possible to observe the progression of the illness. It is common for the problem to regress spontaneously, and suddenly, the hair grows back. In cases where there is severe hair loss, there has been limited success treating alopecia areata with steroids (intradermal, topical, or oral) and other immune modulators such as minoxidil or phototherapy.

External Follicle Hair Loss

Trichotillomania

Trichotillomania (TTM), or "trich," is an impulse control disorder characterized by the repeated urge to pull out scalp and body hair. It may be related distantly to obsessive compulsive disorder (OCD), with which it shares both similarities and differences.

What are the symptoms of trichotillomania?

- Recurrent pulling out of one's hair resulting in noticeable hair loss.
- An increasing sense of tension immediately before pulling out the hair or when resisting the behavior.
- Pleasure, gratification, or relief when pulling out the hair.
- The disturbance is not accounted for by another mental disorder and is not due to a general medical condition (e.g., a dermatological condition).
- The disturbance causes significant distress or impairment in social, occupational, or other important areas of functioning.

How and when does it start?

People often start compulsive hair pulling around the age of 12 to 13, although it is not uncommon for it to start at a much younger or older age. Frequently, a stressful event can be associated with the onset, such as a change of schools, abuse, family conflict, or the death of a parent. The symptoms may also be triggered by pubertal hormonal changes.

Does trichotillomania lead to other problems?

During adolescence—which is an especially crucial time for developing self-esteem, body image, comfort with sexuality, and relationships with peers of both sexes—teens may endure ridicule from family, friends, or classmates in addition to feeling shame over their inability to control the habit. Although many people with trichotillomania successfully overcome the syndrome and go on to live their lives in a normal fashion, including getting married and maintaining rewarding careers, there are those who avoid intimate relationships and any social interaction whatsoever for fear of having their shameful secret exposed.

What is the cause?

There is no specific cause of trichotillomania, but the current thought is that it is a medical illness. On the biological level, one theory is that there is a disruption in the system involving the chemical messengers between the nerve cells in the brain. As with many other illnesses, there may be a combination of factors, such as a genetic predisposition and an aggravating stress or circumstance. Alternatively, trichotillomania could be a symptom caused by different factors in different individuals, just as a cough can be produced by any one of a multitude of medical problems. Finding the cause(s) will take more research.

Habit reversal training

As of this writing, other than medication, the only treatment shown to have any documented effect on the symptoms of trich is a behavioral treatment known as habit reversal training (HRT). This treatment was developed by Dr. Nathan Azrin and his colleagues, and the results were first published in 1973 in the article "Habit Reversal: A Method of Eliminating Nervous Habits and Tics." The treatment focused on getting patients to increase their awareness of their behavior by recording it; learning as much as possible about when, where, and how it occurred; and discovering how to know ahead of time when it would occur. They next were trained to focus on and reduce the tension that preceded the pulling. Finally, they were taught to perform a muscular movement that was inconspicuous, that was the opposite of and incompatible with the behavior they wished to eliminate, and that would become a learned behavior. Many patients who pull their hair don't realize that they are doing this; it is a conditioned response. With HRT, doctors train the individuals to learn to recognize their impulse to pull and also teach them to redirect this impulse. As a part of the behavioral record-keeping component of HRT, patients are often instructed to keep journals of their hair-pulling episodes. They may be asked to record the date, time, location, and number of hairs pulled, as well what they were thinking or feeling at the time. This can help the patient learn to identify situations where they commonly pull out their hair, and develop strategies for avoiding episodes.

My Ground-breaking Research

I have been in the hair industry in some shape or form for more than three decades, during which I have seen women suffer from various types of hair loss. At first, the origins of hair loss perplexed me. For years I, not unlike most in the hair and medical industry, bought into the idea that all hair loss stems from stress, diet, hormones, or some type of genetic alopecia. I had many theories about why women lose hair, and in answer to my prayers for wisdom, I dedicated myself to studying hair loss and was able successfully to develop and prove my theories about hair loss. The results were short hair syndrome (SHS) and follicular epidermis alopecia (FEA).

Research by Trichologists Hooshang and Lisa Akbari

Short hair syndrome (SHS) is the term I coined after years of research and studies. This disorder is, in short, a vicious cycle of hair growth and breakage. SHS prevents the hair strands from obtaining their potential fullness and length. Damage occurs from one or more sources on several areas within a single strand. Hair breakage and loss are the target symptoms and the end results of a group of symptoms that collectively characterize this hair disorder. Also, other related symptoms that will appear within the hair strands are poor elasticity, chronic split ends, layer peeling, changes in hair texture, tears in the hair strands, and, in some cases, slight color changes. Most of these may require a microscopic hair analysis to detect, but some can be discovered through unaided observation.

Follicular epidermis alopecia (FEA) is the name I gave to a form of scalp hair loss that I researched and studied for years. The name is given because the problem occurs in the part of the follicle that rests in the epidermis, and because there is an appearance of alopecia. FEA prevents the hair strand from obtaining length, as areas of the scalp appear to lose the ability to grow hair from particular follicles. This occurs when a blockage around or within the follicle mouth develops, preventing the hair from pushing through the mouth, not allowing the developed shaft to obtain length. A bald appearance on the scalp is the target symptom and the end result along with other symptoms that collectively characterize this hair disorder. Damage to the epidermal scalp and scalp disorders are causes of this type of alopecia. Cosmetic and environmental pollutants perpetually in proximity to the developing hair follicle mouth are the most common causes of this disorder. Furthermore, chronic itch, tenderness, redness, and sore scalp are some of the more common symptoms. Most of these symptoms may require a microscopic hair analysis to detect, but some can be discovered through unaided observation. Although FEA is quite often misdiagnosed as FPB, the two are very different. FEA occurs in the epidermal (outer) layer of the scalp where the follicle mouth rests. FBP occurs in the dermis (inner) layer of the scalp where the hair follicle rests.

SHS and FEA are both categorized as forms of external follicle hair loss and are predominately found in women, but they can also occur in men and children. Women unknowingly tend to do more negative things to their scalps and hair surfaces when manipulating their hair. Although both SHS and FEA can develop on any area of the head, I have found that the crown is the number one area, and the hairline is the number two area. In some cases, advanced levels of SHS or FEA dominate most of the scalp. In extreme cases, the damage can even cause a complete loss of visible scalp hair. Most women suffer from some level of SHS and FEA, so I strongly recommend you reread this chapter, taking notes, and then contact your stylist or a trichologist to see if you need to take action to save your beautiful hair.

Why Is My Hair Becoming Thinner?

In this section, you will learn about layer peeling and strand separation, which cause a texture change resulting in strand thinning. The life of a single strand can be a dangerous one, especially with the abuse that some of us put our strands through. If your strands knew what the future held for them and how they would be treated, and if they had a choice, they would never surface! Many women think that their hair and scalp problems happen all of a sudden, but there is a process that leads to damage.

As a single strand ages, it literally can fall apart layer by layer before it dies away or breaks off. Hair is resilient, as it deals with damage, but as SHS develops, the cuticle will peel away and the strand will begin to separate. As the cortical fibers become exposed, the hair loses its elasticity and some parts of the strand break away. As the aging damage continues and the disorder progresses, you may notice that, although your hair has some length, the hair does not seem as full or your ponytails seem thinner than they once were. This is called a texture change: your strands have become smaller than their normal size. As you have learned, texture deals with the size of your strand, and a texture change means that your strand is getting smaller. At this point, strand thinning, which is a form of SHS, has occurred. If your strands continue to lose cuticle layers, then they will not have enough elasticity to support simple combing and parting; the hair will die or break. As SHS develops into a more advanced stage, you will notice areas of short hair throughout your head.

This form of aging damage, resulting in SHS, can occur in any life cycle of a strand that the follicle produces. Now, let's talk for a minute about how all this happens. The number one cause of SHS is chemical damage, and the number two cause is pressured heat. If a chemical is applied to your strand and is left on longer than your strand can tolerate, the strand begins to swell and expose its inner layers as the outer layers separate and peel, until the strand finally breaks away. With excessive pressured heat, your layers begin to melt away on the surface. While all this is going on, your strands are getting smaller and smaller, then shorter and shorter. Such is the fate of your luscious locks when strand thinning sets in. Ask questions about any chemicals used on your hair, and find alternatives to pressured heat to avoid this tragic fate.

CHAPTER SEVEN:

WILL TRIMMING MAKE MY HAIR GROW FASTER?

In this chapter, you will learn that you have a choice to either treat or trim your hair. I'll also tell you how to make a responsible choice, letting you know when to treat and when to trim and why.

"My stylist said that I should trim my hair. Is that a good idea?" "Will trimming my hair help my hair grow?" Those are the two main questions that I am asked, to which I always give the same answer. You have two options in dealing your split ends: to trim or to treat.

In my days as a stylist and for many years afterward, I believed that trimming my clients' ends would help their hair to grow, which was an insane contradiction. If I trimmed her ends, then I would be taking away hair length. I knew that hair grows from the scalp and not from the shaft, but, like many stylists today, I convinced my clients that this removal of dead ends was just a part of growing hair. Split ends come from wear, tear, and aging damage. If the ends are not cut, the split ends will peel into the remainder of the hair shaft. When this happens, the hair loses its ability to obtain length, so it seems like common sense to believe that your hair won't grow unless you trim the ends. The fact is, trimming your ends will not make your hair grow longer, and to say that it will just is not the truth. Cutting your hair makes your hair shorter; therefore, each time your hair is trimmed, some of your length is lost.

But the question still needs to be answered: should you trim your ends or not? The answer is yes and no. You have two options in dealing with split ends; you can treat them or not; if you decide not to treat them, then you should cut them. The choice is entirely yours, but remember, you must choose one or the other. If you choose not to cut your ends, you must choose to treat them, or eventually they will peel away the strand. When the strand peels away, you still will have the problem obtaining length, and you still will feel that your hair is not growing.

Ask yourself why you are having your hair trimmed. Ends should be cut for two reasons: for grooming purposes or to remove damaged hair. If you want certain hairstyles, your stylist may not be able to achieve them without trimming your hair. My advice to you is to stay assertive, be involved, and be reasonable. Make clear to your stylist your goals for your hair. Most important, remember, you can treat or you can trim. You can do either, but you can't do neither!

Chapter Eight:

How Can I Get a Younger Scalp?

In this chapter, you will learn how to create a clean, acidic, stimulated, hydrated environment for your hair and why it is an important part in an anti-aging process. I will also share with you my personal stability program to best help your scalp regain its youth.

The important lesson of this chapter is, keep your scalp clean, acidic, stimulated, and hydrated in order to keep it healthy. You know now that your scalp is skin, and you know also that your skin can and will age. The big question is how you can slow down the aging of your scalp. A closely related question is why it is important to stop accelerated aging of your scalp.

First, let's talk about why it is important. The scalp is the foundation of hair growth because hair is an appendage of the scalp, and if your scalp is not protected and preserved on a constant basis, then aging damage will occur, ultimately causing hair loss. You can prevent aging damage and have a scalp half its age by creating a certain environment. It is simple, and you won't need medicine or expensive treatments if you commit yourself to following a few simple rules.

Pollutants

Pollutants are contaminants that can become toxic. Over time, this turns out to be detrimental to the overall health of the scalp. Pollutants create a home for pathogens, disease-causing bacteria that can live, breed, and grow on the scalp. There are three categories of pollutants that contribute to scalp aging, causing scalp disorders and potentially causing permanent hair loss.

Scalp Pollutants

Scalp pollutants develop when the dead skin cells that shed from the epidermis are trapped in the hair follicle mouth. The scalp is like the rest of the body and sheds dead cells on a continual basis as a natural part of renewing the skin. Dead cells on our body fall away easily from bathing and showering, being brushed away by our clothing, or just seem to dissipate into the air. Dead scalp cells are trapped by our hair and, after a period of time, settle into the scalp pores, including the hair follicle mouth. After about three days of scalp shedding, the dead epidermal cells begin to build up, clogging the pores and becoming pollutants that cause aging damage.

Environmental Pollutants

Environmental pollutants develop when dust, dirt, debris, pollen, and other such things in the air collect in your hair. Once all of these get into the hair, over a few days, they work their way to the scalp, becoming trapped on the hair and in the scalp pores. Even if you spend most of your time indoors, you cannot escape the dust, pet dander, and other pollutants in your home or place of work.

Cosmetic Pollutants

Cosmetic pollutants can develop when we use certain scalp and hair products to style our hair. One problem is that many of the most popular products are not water soluble—they don't break down well in water—so even if you shampoo often, certain hair and scalp products won't rinse clean or shampoo away easily. Products that contain wax, grease, and certain fillers will clog the scalp pores and leave a filmy negative buildup on the hair. Also, if you use conditioning or moisturizing shampoos, they will leave traces of the product on the hair and scalp.

Clarifying Your Scalp

Scalp, environmental, and cosmetic pollutants can cause aging damage to the hair and scalp. Let me make an analogy to explain. Think about what happens to the pores on your face when they become clogged. Aging damage will occur in many ways, including dehydration, bumps, and many other skin problems, which is one of the reasons why we have facials. Think about what we do in order to unclog the pores on the face. One of the first steps in all anti-aging treatments is to clean the pores. Accordingly, your scalp and hair should be cleaned with a clarifying shampoo that has a pH between 4.5 and 5.5. A clarified scalp will aid in resisting some scalp diseases and relieve some scalp problems such as itchy, flaky, and even tender scalp. Clarifying hair won't remove all of the pollutants that cause scalp problems, but it will enable your conditioner to work better, giving body to your hair. Overall, you clarify your hair and scalp in order to protect and preserve hair and scalp fitness, which is the first step in an anti-aging plan.

Another crucial part of an anti-aging treatment is to always keep your scalp in a clean, acidic, stimulated, hydrated environment. Allow me to break down the different elements of that environment so it will be more understandable and so that you can create this nourishing environment for your hair.

A Clean Environment

This rule is most important and is mandatory in an anti-aging treatment for the scalp. Let's examine more closely the number one rule of creating a clean environment. One question that I am asked often is, "How often should I shampoo?" My answer is always the same, "Shampoo your hair and scalp on an as-needed basis." To be more specific, you should shampoo at least every three days, possibly more often depending on how active you are and your scalp type. But you should never go longer than a week without shampooing your scalp. If you have an oily scalp, you may need to shampoo every day and, in some cases, twice a day. If you work out or experience scalp sweats, you should shampoo every other day or, in some cases, every day. You must also keep in mind that you should have a special scalp care regimen in cases when you may have a scalp disorder.

By clarifying and creating a clean environment on your scalp, you will prevent negative buildups from forming, because they prevent the follicle mouth and entire scalp from becoming polluted. Recall the three categories of pollutants and the dangers of allowing them to settle on the scalp.

An Acidic Environment

Your shampoo should be acid-based; that is, it should be within the range of the pH of your scalp, which is 4.5 to 5.5. This will keep your scalp in its natural balance and free you from the fear of shampooing. Many women are afraid that if they shampoo as often as recommended or needed, they will cause damage to both their hair and scalps. My studies have shown the reason for this fear is that women commonly use the wrong shampoos, with the wrong pH level. Because shampoo is the product that has the most direct contact with your scalp, you must be careful in making your choice. You will need a mildly acidic clarifying shampoo with a pH level between 4.5 and 5.5. By doing so, you will not disturb the basic chemistry of the scalp, allowing you to shampoo as often as you like. When you use a shampoo outside of the range of your scalp pH, your scalp will itch, flake, and become dry. Also, you should never use a conditioning shampoo, because they have fillers and softening agents that, while making the hair feel soft, will cause a filmy buildup on the scalp. It is impossible to clean and condition your hair and scalp at the same time! Think about it, can you bathe and put on lotion at the same time? Obviously, you can't. Therefore, neither can you use shampoo and conditioner at the same time. The bottom line is, there are no real benefits to using a conditioning or moisturizing shampoo; with the one, your scalp and hair are not getting clean, period, end of discussion.

A Stimulated Environment

Scalp is skin, and skin is an organ; like all organs, it functions better and benefits from good blood circulation. We also must keep in mind that the scalp houses the hair follicle, and each follicle is a tiny organ with arteries and veins attached to them; thus, scalp stimulation is a crucial part of a scalp anti-aging program. You should stimulate your scalp each day. In some cases, when you may have a tight scalp due to holding tension in your scalp, you should stimulate it twice a day. If you are experiencing hair loss, you will benefit greatly from scalp stimulation.

Massage your scalp while shampooing by sliding your fingers under your hair and placing the balls of your fingers on the scalp to deeply massage or rub the scalp. Remember, you must never scratch your scalp with your fingernails, shampoo brush, or any other object, because it will create tears on the scalp that will lead to further damage. Remember also that you should never rub a dry scalp, because that will wear away the top epidermal layers of the scalp, making the scalp sensitive and vulnerable to damage. The reason it is safe to rub your scalp during shampooing is that your fingers are able to glide and slide over the scalp because your scalp is completely wet, and the shampoo acts as a lubricant.

There is a safe way to stimulate your scalp other than when you are shampooing. First, make yourself comfortable while sitting at a table. Place your elbows on the table, and then put your head in your hands by placing one hand on the right side of your head and the other on the left. Press your hands and fingers against your scalp while moving the skin back and forth. Repeat ten times, both horizontally and vertically, while taking deep breaths. This scalp exercise can be done almost anywhere, as long as you are comfortable, have a flat surface, and are able to take deep breaths.

A Hydrated Environment

Your scalp can become dry or dehydrated for many reasons. Medications, chemicals, and hair products are a few of the culprits. A dehydrated scalp will cause scalp aging and ultimately can cause hair loss. Your top epidermal cells naturally hold moisture, so the key to hydrating a dry scalp is to seal the natural moisture in. If you suffer from dry scalp, you will need to seal the scalp while it is clean and slightly moist. You can do this by applying an oil—not a grease (a grease is heavier)—to your scalp after rinsing with conditioner. Simply blot the scalp to remove the excess water, and then lightly glaze it using an oil. Also, if you have dry scalp and fine hair, apply the oil on your scalp and leave it on while your hair is conditioned under a warm dryer. Next, rinse it away with very warm water. Check that the oil will rinse completely from the scalp and hair each time you shampoo. To be sure that the oil is not a grease product and won't clog your pores, apply a small amount on the back of your hand and rinse your hand with warm, forceful water. The oil should dissolve and rinse easily; a grease product will leave a filmy buildup on the skin and thus will not be scalp-friendly. Keep your scalp clean, acidic, hydrated, and stimulated in order to keep it healthy and young.

Unclogging Scalp Pores

Unclogged scalp pores have many anti-aging benefits, and I recommend that you follow the steps I've laid out for you at least every season change, possibly more often depending on how active you are, if you have scalp problems, or if your hair and scalp are exposed to scalp, environmental, or cosmetic pollutants on a regular basis. When your pores are clean and clear, your scalp feels better, like it is breathing—remember, scalp is skin, and it must be allowed to breathe. Scalp itch, tenderness, and other problems will go away. In my clinic, I use a treatment of deep cleaning and detoxifying the scalp in cases of chronically clogged pores, using in-clinic treatment products and specially trained scalp therapists. I conducted a study to create a home program that will give you similar results. You can begin to unclog your scalp pores by following a few simple steps. The initial condition of your scalp will determine how long it will take to see results. If you follow my instructions to the letter, you will notice a positive change, namely, your scalp regaining its youth!

Cleansing Program

Before you begin, you need to get ready by gathering some supplies:
- A cleansing, clarifying, and balancing shampoo (always use a scalp- and hair-friendly clarifying shampoo)
- An applicator bottle that has a narrow but not sharp tip, as well as a cap
- A plastic cap for your head
- Long strips of cotton
- A tabletop dryer or heat cap
- Lots of very warm, forcefully running water (the shower is usually the best)

Note: I recommend my cleansing, clarifying, and balancing shampoo, which I formulated to clean and clarify with mild agents that work without stripping your hair. This shampoo purifies both your hair and scalp by putting them in a pure, natural state. Most importantly, I did not add conditioning or moisturizing fillers to my shampoo, because they cause cosmetic pollutants to develop. Finally, I carefully balanced the pH to keep your hair's natural level of 4.5 to 5.5.

Now that you've gathered all of your supplies, let's begin!

Start by preheating your dryer for ten minutes on high. By the way, this is the one time you should preheat your dryer before use. You must be careful, if you choose a heat cap, not to burn your scalp. Next, pour the clarifying shampoo into the applicator bottle. Shampoo your hair and scalp generously, parting your hair with the tip of the applicator cap as you do so. After you have applied the shampoo, place your fingers on your scalp being sure to slide your fingers under hair to reach the scalp. Massage your scalp, focusing on any problem areas. Next, rub the shampoo throughout your hair. Place cotton around your hairline and the plastic cap on your head. Sit under the preheated dryer for ten minutes; you should be sweating. If you don't sweat easily, then sit for at least fifteen minutes. Next, using very warm, forcefully running water, rinse all areas of your scalp, again focusing on problem areas.

How do your hair and scalp feel? Pretty good, I'll bet, fresh and clean. But wait! You've only just begun; you successfully have prepared your hair for the treatment program. Allow me to outline the basic steps of that program for you.

Treatment Program

1. Shampoo and rinse your hair and scalp in two more applications of a cleansing, clarifying, and balancing shampoo.

2. Condition your hair using a deep-penetrating, moisturizing, and stabilizing conditioner.

3. Towel-blot your hair by squeezing the strands carefully; never handle your hair roughly.

4. Part your hair and apply the conditioner in a downward direction toward the strand ends. Place a plastic cap on your head and sit under a warm dryer for ten minutes.

5. Remove the plastic cap and carefully rinse your hair, sliding your fingers in a downward direction with warm water. Be sure to use very warm, forceful water on your scalp. Rinsing is important! Also make sure to apply a leave-in conditioner.

6. Towel-blot your scalp and hair, squeezing your hair to remove excess water. Spray hair vitamins throughout your hair, paying special attention to the strands.

7. Apply oil sheen in a jar to your scalp immediately after you towel-blot and spray your hair. By doing so, you will seal in the natural hydration from your already slightly moistened scalp.

In this chapter, you have learned how to create a clean, acidic, stimulated, hydrated environment and why it is an important part of an anti-aging treatment. You are aware of the three categories of pollutants, as well as how to unclog scalp pores and stop the development of such on your scalp and hair. Now that I've given you the education, it is your job to continue learning, as well as to memorize these basic steps. Most importantly, you must actually perform the basic steps and the clarifying treatment to keep your scalp young and healthy, now and for years to come.

Chapter Nine:

What Do I Need to Know about Treatment?

In this chapter, you will learn how and when to give special treatment to your scalp and hair in order to stabilize any problems. For example, protect your hair from the dryer by rotating the rollers and by applying oil the scalp while your hair is wet. To protect your hair from outside dryness, apply moisturizer to your hair before going into a dry environment. I will tell you how to maintain the recovery that is achieved during the stabilization treatments. For example, you will learn how to balance the delicate protein and moisture levels within the hair shaft to prevent the strand from aging, and why it is important to do so. Additionally, I'll share with you my knowledge of how to prevent hair and scalp problems from returning, which slows down the process against hair aging.

Preventing Aging Damage

A large percentage of women who are losing hair have a form of aging loss where the hair literally is falling apart, and in some cases, the damage is beyond repair. But in many cases, with the proper treatment, you will be able to mend the hair to stop the symptom of hair breakage. Since any form of hair loss can be very traumatic, I believe that a woman should have the option to save her hair if at all possible. But I also believe if the damage is extreme to the point that it is beyond repair, you may want to simply cut the damaged hair away. Keep in mind that the hair will grow back, and the new hair will stay youthful as long as you protect and preserve the strands. In my clinic, I offer the option to treat the hair problems of many women, and the one thing that most have in common is that they want the treatment in order to stop the problems, but they don't want to change their damaging habits. In other words, they want me to help them, but they want to attach all of their "I can'ts" and "I won'ts" to the program that I put together for them. Every day I hear, "I can't stop doing this," or "I won't give up that," or "I will not do this." I often have to remind them that there was a process that brought about the damage, and there will be a process that brings about the healing. Frequently, I hear some of my clients say that their hair "all of a sudden just started falling out," and I have to explain that this was not "all of a sudden."

The process of aging damage is, in many cases, a slow process. Think of how you feel as your body ages. If you have not taken very good care of your body, you feel as if you are falling apart. Well, when your strands begin aging, each strand really will fall apart. First, the hair strand becomes dry and brittle, and then, layer by layer, the strand peels away until the elasticity becomes so poor that there is not enough elasticity to support simply combing your hair. The hair falls out, even when you just touch it. My programs are designed in three parts: to treat the scalp and hair, when needed, in order to stabilize any problems; to maintain the recovery that is achieved through stabilization treatments; and to prevent problems from returning or even occurring in the first place. This three-part program of stabilization, maintenance, and prevention will slow down the aging process and will enable your hair to remain on your head for its entire life cycle.

When your hair and scalp become damaged, you must give them special treatment in order to stabilize any problems. Recovery requires a change in the way you treat your hair. It will not be necessary for you to change your style, give up chemicals, or even give up heated styling tools forever. But in order to stabilize any problems, you will need to create a consistent environment for your hair and scalp. This may mean that you have to stop using some of those chemicals or heated tools for a while, until your problems are stable, before reintroducing them. It is crucial for recovery that you are willing to change and do things in a safe, anti-aging manner.

Part One: Stabilization

Depending on the extent of the aging damage, part one could last for four, seven, or twelve weeks. In some rare cases, it can take as long as six months to stabilize a problem. The key is to stick with it. Think of your hair as a person in a hospital critical care unit. That person must be watched over and cared for very closely, and all medicines and treatments must be delivered consistently. With stabilization treatments, your hair must have a similar type of program in order to recover. Let's pretend you are one of my clients. You are suffering from SHS and are experiencing chronic breakage. You tell me that your hair "just won't grow." You have new growth on the scalp level, but your hair "grows to a certain length and then stops growing." I recommend twelve weeks to stabilize. During stabilization our goal is to stop your hair from breaking so that we can move into part two: maintenance. Weeks one through twelve will follow the stabilizing program that is very similar to the basic treatment described in Chapter 8.

You should shampoo following this stabilizing program every two days. Remember that it is important to balance your hair and scalp by keeping the natural pH of 4.5 to 5.5. Also remember that using a leave-in conditioner and hair vitamins are vital in treating SHS.

Conditioning is slightly different for stabilizing hair. Use a deep-penetrating, protein moisturizing, and stabilizing conditioner, which is an intensive conditioning agent that naturally repairs, rebuilds, and rejuvenates hair. Towel-blot your hair by carefully squeezing strands. Never handle your hair roughly. Next, part your hair and apply conditioner to the ends, scalp hair, and throughout. It is important that you focus on the weak areas. Also, do not comb the conditioner into your hair; instead, carefully rub your hair starting from the top of your head. Place a plastic cap on your head and sit under a warm dryer for ten minutes. Then, remove the plastic cap, apply more conditioner to the ends, and sit back under the dryer for ten more minutes. Next, remove the plastic cap and apply conditioner to your hair closest to the scalp; sit back under the dryer for ten more minutes, for a total of thirty minutes. Finally, remove the plastic cap and carefully rinse by sliding your fingers down the strands with warm water. Be sure to hold a very warm and strong water force close to the scalp. As always, rinsing is important.

Hair vitamins aid in stabilizing the breakage by filling the torn and thin areas of the hair shaft, thus improving the elasticity of your hair. Breakage stops as the strands mend. Part your hair and spray hair vitamins on the ends and weak areas, as well as around the hairline, and throughout your hair.

During the stabilization period, you should avoid all heated tools; roller-setting is a better option. Apply drops of a sculpting lotion to your hair, and then proceed with set-on rollers. Do not blow dry, curl, press, or use a flat iron on your hair at this time.

Styling during Stabilization

This area is a crossroads for many women as they go through stabilization, because they find themselves in a situation where they have to make a very important decision. I am talking about their willingness to do whatever it takes and whatever is needed in order to stabilize their hair problems.

I have treated the damaged hair of many women for many years, and the problem is almost always the same. Most women put hairstyle before hair care, not necessarily intentionally, but nonetheless, it is their reality. When they are in situations where they must choose treatment over style, many women, believe it or not, find this a hard pill to swallow. In my clinic, as I counsel and make recommendations, many clients say to me that they want their problems to go away, but that it is crucial they be able to keep their hair, and I quote, "looking decent"—that is, looking good all the time. My answer to them is the same I am going to give to you: "It may not be possible."

Let me explain. Your hair is damaged, weak, and breaking off. As I mentioned earlier, think of your hair as a sick person who is in the hospital's critical care unit. If that person does not get the care she needs in order to get better, then she may die. Because we definitely do not want that, she must hold off doing the things she normally does or looking the way she normally looks until she heals. This means for you, that if you don't stop and give your hair the care it needs in order to stabilize the problems, it surely will die away before its time. You need to understand and accept that sick hair cannot and will not look normal or as decent as you may like it to look during this fragile period. During this stabilization time, you will be able to style your hair, but it may not be the way that you normally wear your hair. However, all is not lost; you very well will be able to have a nice style that will make you feel comfortable when you go out each day. Stabilization doesn't have to mean boring and bland. Be safe, but have fun and be creative!

First, let's think about things you shouldn't do while you are going through the stabilization process, and then I will give you some options for things you can do for styling.

Don't do

When your hair is breaking away, you need to stop using all heated styling tools because your cuticle layers, the top protective layers, of the strands are weak, torn, lifting, and wearing away. At this time, heated tools will only aggravate an existing problem. Your strands need healthy cuticles in order to tolerate the direct pressured heat that is administered by heated tools such as blow dryers and curling irons.

Also, during the first four to seven weeks of the stabilization of your hair problems and, in some cases, all twelve weeks, you must avoid all chemical services. Now, I know some of you are thinking that I must be out of my mind, that there is no way you will last that long. But before you "chemoholics," or addicts of chemical hair treatments, forget: this is a do-or-die situation for your hair! And don't worry, I will throw you a lifeline when we get to the "can do" section. Remember, in order to stabilize your problems, you must create a consistent, healthy, and healing environment for your hair and scalp for a period of time. Hair chemicals and heated tools will disrupt the new environment that you are attempting to create. If you reintroduce chemicals or heated tools too soon, you will find yourself with a series of small setbacks and eventually convince yourself that the treatment process did not work for you. Later, I will teach you how to reintroduce heated tools and chemicals, except this time you will be empowered to use them in a safe manner.

Can do

You could wear a hairpiece, such as a wig, during this time. I know many of you may have never worn one or, if you have tried them before, don't like wigs. However, wearing a wig is a sure way to take care of your style issue. Think of it as a new look or a way to temporarily change your look. Go to a wig store and try on some of the styles; just remember to start with styles and colors that are similar to what you are accustomed to. Many ladies who have gone through my treatment programs at first hated the ideas of wigs, but then after their hair was better, and even when they resumed styling their natural hair, they reported that, from time to time, they wore their wigs for fun or for a change. They also told me that they got a lot of compliments from friends. In Chapter 10, I will teach you how to safely wear wigs and other added hair.

Apply a moisturizer each day to maintain hydration. In order to retain the moisture levels in your hair, you, like many women, will need a support product like moisturizer for your new hair growth. Then, lightly apply oil to seal in hydration. If your hair is over-processed or thin, you may not have the cuticle layers to support oil or moisturizer; that is, when you apply it, your hair will become limp. If this is the case, use just a small amount of oil or moisturizer, and you should be fine. A real treat that I recommend for any condition of hair is to sleep on a satin pillow case.

Here's the lifeline I promised to replace heated tools: roller-set your hair instead. Also, replace gel and mousse products with a sculpting lotion to set hair or to lay down the hairline. Sit under the dryer for ten minutes for short hair, twenty minutes for medium hair, or thirty minutes for long hair, rotating rollers every five to ten minutes. If your hair is not dry, let it dry naturally afterward. Don't forget to sip on cool water while under the dryer to prevent sweating. Alternatively, sometimes you simply can use a leave-in conditioner and let your hair dry naturally.

Part Two: Maintenance

A maintenance program should be followed for six months to a year, depending on how well your hair and scalp stabilized. Maintenance means your problems are stable; in other words, your hair should feel more hydrated, and breakage should be slowing down or, at this stage, even stopping. In this part, we are going to focus on maintaining the recovery that you achieved during stabilization. Some women get a false sense of security during the maintenance stage, because their hair and scalps feel and look so much better from when they began this three-step healing program. You must remember that at this point, you are only just out of the critical stage; your problems are stable, but your hair is not well yet. Therefore, the maintenance program is a very important step in renewing the youth of your hair and should be followed accordingly.

During maintenance, you will be able to achieve your desired length of hair. Another good thing I know you'll want to hear about this stage is that you should be able to reintroduce chemicals and semipermanent rinses. The key to safely using chemicals without over-processing your new healthy hair is to chemically treat only the new hair growth. For curly hair, never relax your hair until you have enough new natural growth so that your stylist can see a clear line of difference between the natural scalp hair and the previously relaxed hair, which should have been relaxed no earlier than eight weeks ago, even though ten weeks would be optimal. For straight hair, never get a permanent wave on previously permed hair. You can get a root perm, but no sooner than two months after successfully stabilizing your hair.

The same rule applies to any permanent color and any other chemical treatments. If you make a habit of applying and reapplying permanent chemicals and colors to previously treated hair, you will eventually end up back in the predicament of having over-processed, aging hair and scalp damage. Always treat your hair and scalp gently when reintroducing chemicals and permanent rinses; it is best to err on the side of caution. That is why you still shouldn't use heated tools until all of your older, damaged hair has been grown out and cut away. Instead, continue to roller-set your hair or just wear it naturally.

After completing stabilization, for the next six to twelve months you should follow the maintenance program, which is very simple because it is only slightly different from the stabilization program. For the maintenance program, repeat the shampooing steps of the stabilization program at least twice a week or more often, depending on how active you are. Remember to rinse your hair and scalp with very warm, forceful water.

Next, condition your hair with a deep-penetrating, protein moisturizing, and stabilizing conditioner. Be careful to towel-blot your hair by squeezing the strands gently; never handle your hair roughly. Part your hair and apply conditioner to the ends and throughout. It is important not to comb your hair to spread the conditioner. Instead, carefully rub your hair starting from the top of your head. Put on a plastic cap and sit under a warm dryer for five minutes. Afterward, remove the plastic cap and apply more conditioner to your ends and sit back under the dryer for five more minutes. Remove the cap and massage the conditioner that is on your hair, hairline, and throughout; sit under the dryer for five more minutes, for a total of fifteen minutes. Remove the cap and carefully rinse your hair by sliding your fingers down the strands and using very warm water. Be sure to hold a strong water force close to your scalp.

After you rinse out the moisturizing conditioner, towel-blot your hair to dry. Be sure to squeeze out any excess water. A leave-in conditioner and hair vitamins will aid in protecting the hair shaft, thus keeping the porosity and elasticity of your hair even. Part your hair and spray hair vitamins on your ends, hairline, and throughout your hair. To style your hair, apply drops of a sculpting lotion and proceed with set-on rollers. Alternatively, you can let your hair dry naturally and then style by lightly applying oil to your scalp after your hair is dry.

Part Three: Prevention

Prevention is the stage that we all love, because the prevention stage means your hair and scalp are well and no longer sick. You can breathe and be relieved that your hair and scalp have returned to a youthful state and are no longer suffering from the effect of aging damage. Now, before you get too comfortable and ride off into the sunset of healthy hair bliss, there are some things that you need to know. The prevention program, unlike the others, isn't followed for simply a few weeks. It is a lifetime change: never returning to old, bad, thoughtless habits that got you into trouble in the first place. You will need to follow this program from now on in order to prevent hair and scalp problems from returning. The prevention program will slow down the hair aging process and keep you from losing hair other than through natural shedding. Now, isn't just the thought of that enough to make you want to shout for joy?

Your prevention program should include a plan that you can put faithfully into action, because this is about life change. Don't become stressed out, just relax and apply the knowledge that you have gained by reading *Every Woman's Guide to Beautiful Hair at Any Age*. Think about your hair the same way you do your body. When you want to maintain health, you follow a regimen and a lifestyle that are conducive to good health. Well, you are going to do the same for your hair—without stress—so that your hair can reap the benefits of good, sound care. Your prevention program should be designed to fit your lifestyle and should be adjusted depending on your reality. In other words, your program should not be too rigid or strict, just consistent.

Apply the same basic rules about chemicals and heated tools that I have taught you throughout this guide. Remember to shampoo and condition your hair on a regular basis, shampooing as often as needed, depending on how active you are, and deep conditioning twice a week or at least once a week. Don't think that you can get by doing anything sporadically. Also remember that there is a process to aging hair damage, and it does not happen overnight. Your aging hair problems will return to remind you if you forget this.

And just remember, if you find yourself in a situation where you have damaged your hair beyond repair and your hair is going through a slow death, one that is causing you to go through torturous anxiety, give yourself permission to cut your hair off and start over. But first, take a long hard look in the mirror and make mental and physical notes, and perhaps take a picture. Record the events leading up to the hair disaster. Now promise that person in the mirror that you will never repeat this hair crime again. Okay now lighten up; no condemnation, only conviction and a commitment to change is required.

CHAPTER TEN:

CAN I AND SHOULD I ADD HAIR? AND HOW?

In this chapter, you will learn how to throw caution to the wind (safely), have some fun, and look like a movie star. I will tell you about all types of added hair, temporary and not so temporary, and ways to extend your hair length or fullness using hair weaves, lace front wigs, and other hair attachments. I'll share with you what is easy and what is not, what are the pros and cons, and how to know which hair attachment is right for you. Most importantly, you will discover how to enjoy wearing added hair without causing aging damage to your hair or scalp.

Added hair can be a beautiful expression of image and style and can be used by anyone. You should be free to make the decision to add hair, but you must know how to do it in a safe manner in order to prevent hair and scalp damage. With many hair attachments, what starts out as a good thing soon turns into a bad thing. In other words, before you make the decision to add new hair in any shape, form, or fashion, I am sure you envision a beautiful new adventure that perhaps may bring sex appeal, fun, and even freedom. But instead, you end up with something unexpected and what seems to be a never-ending nightmare.

Remember to stay assertive and pay close attention to what is being done to your hair. Added hair does not have to be painful, and when it is removed, your hair should have some added length with fullness.

Before actually adding hair, be sure to set aside some time and request counseling with an expert; remember to ask complete questions and wait for complete answers. Also, keep in mind that many of these professionals usually are very busy and may seem arrogant. For courage, tell yourself that you are paying them, and you always can go somewhere else. Don't be intimidated; no question is a dumb one. I advise that, before and after your counseling, you do some research on the type of added hair you are interested in and research the one that you and your stylist have decided on. Added hair is something that can be enjoyed at any age. The first thing you should do is decide on the style you want, then seek out an expert, for example, in hair weaving or braiding. I can guarantee that you will not enjoy your weave or braids if you don't do your research.

Hair Weaves

Hair weaving is a process of adding a hair-like extension to your natural hair to obtain length or fullness. Experts are coming up with new ways of adding hair all the time. Some of the basic and most common ways are bonding or sewing added hair using various creative techniques. Unfortunately, this causes many women to suffer damage to their hair and scalps. Added hair can wind up being a good thing gone bad. But if you are assertive in selecting an excellent stylist, your hair and scalp will not suffer.

Bonding

The most important thing to remember when bonding is, added hair should not be bonded to your scalp. This can cause serious scalp damage that eventually will lead to scalp disorders and hair loss. If the mouth of the follicle is bonded in any way, it will trap all categories of pollutants within it and literally smother the scalp. When the follicle mouth is hot bonded, your scalp may be burned. Additionally, when the bonded hair is removed, it will pull away some or all of your epidermal cells, taking some of your hair with them, which can result in serious balding, as well as cause scalp damage. It is important to add bonded hair only strand to strand or hair to hair, and never to the scalp.

There are two main ways to add hair by bonding: cold glue or hot glue. Cold glue is a bonding adhesive that is applied cold to hair wefts or strands that are then applied to your hair. Hot glue, better known as hair infusion, is a bonding adhesive that is loaded into a glue gun and applied hot to hair wefts or strands that are then applied to your hair. Both hot and cold bonding should be used only for temporarily added hair. These types of attachments can be worn safely, without scalp or hair damage, for up to three months if shampooed and conditioned at least every three days. All bonding adhesives should be removed with the proper adhesive remover; do not take any shortcuts and try to remove them using something you found at home. The proper remover should allow your hair to slide away easily without any tugging. If tugging and pulling occurs, you will cause aging damage to your hair cuticle layers, causing the strand elasticity to become poor, and hair breakage will occur. Ultimately, your strands will develop SHS. If your hair is tugged or pulled when the bonding is removed, it means that either the wrong remover is being used or you have not allowed enough time for the remover to soften the adhesive.

Sewing

There are various ways a weave can be sewn in. In most cases your natural hair is braided flat to your scalp, then, with a needle, a weft of hair is sewn into your braided hair. The most important thing to remember when having a weave sewn in is to be sure your scalp is not pulled, because this will cause scalp damage and even hair loss. The weft of hair should be sewn tightly to attach it securely to the braid, but should not be tugging at your scalp. Also, you must be sure that the professional is using a dull-tipped needle so that he or she does not poke or puncture your scalp.

Braids

Braiding is a process of creating various plaits using added hair. In some cases, your own hair can be used as well. Many women who opt for braids suffer from aging damage to their scalps and hair for two main reasons. The number one reason is that most braiders pull the hair too tightly as they are braiding, and the hair follicle mouth becomes torn and enlarged. This damage will result in scalp infections and hair loss, particularly at the hairline. You can wear braids without damage by making sure that your braids are attached in a safe manner. The same thing applies with braids as it does with weaves: the braid should not be tight at the scalp. The number two reason is that many women don't think they have to care for their scalps and hair as they normally would, while wearing braids. Commonly, women won't shampoo and condition on a regular basis, and the scalp and hair become polluted and dehydrated. Not only does this cause aging damage, it also weakens your natural hair. After the braids are removed, your hair is broken or will begin to fall away after a few short weeks. I have seen women with less hair than they started with before braiding! But this doesn't have to happen to you. You can enjoy your braids without causing aging damage, hair loss, or scalp problems by following the proper care program. Remember: braids are low-maintenance hairstyles and not *zero-maintenance* styles!

Caring for Weaves and Braids

In order to have a healthy scalp and healthy hair while wearing added hair, you must follow a care program to the letter. I created this special program that is highly effective but surprisingly simple.

You should wash your hair with a cleansing, clarifying, and balancing shampoo every four to seven days or even more often depending how active you are. Rinse your hair for one to three minutes with warm water, holding the water close to your scalp. Apply more shampoo, parting the added hair with your fingers and massaging the in-between areas. Also, massage the shampoo into any itchy or flaky areas, being careful not to scratch your scalp with your nails. Rub down the added hair toward the ends. Do not rub or push the added hair up into scalp.

Rinse again, holding the water close to your scalp between the added hair. Remember to rinse your hairline and behind your ears. Reapply shampoo to your moistened hair and scalp; this time let shampoo sit for one minute. Finally, rinse a final time, making sure to clean your scalp, natural hair, and added hair thoroughly.

Using a towel, blot your scalp between the added hair. Then blot down the added hair. Apply a deep-penetrating, protein moisturizing, and stabilizing conditioner to your hairline and the part of added hair that is closest to your scalp. Next, rub the conditioner down the added hair toward the ends. Place a plastic cap on your head and sit under a warm dryer for ten minutes. Remove the plastic cap and apply more conditioner to your scalp and the base of the added hair. Sit back under the dryer for ten minutes more. Remove the cap and apply conditioner to the added hair. Rinse with warm water, first holding the water force close to your scalp between the added hair and then down the added hair. Be sure that all of the conditioner is removed; repeat if needed.

Towel-blot your scalp between the added hair and your hairline, then squeeze and blot down the added hair, removing as much water as possible. Apply a leave-in conditioner to the base of the added hair as well as to your hairline. Spray hair vitamins to your hairline, the base of the added hair, and down the added hair toward the ends. Next, apply a moisturizer to your hairline and the base of the added hair. Finally, rub oil on your scalp between the added hair and hairline. Each night before bed, apply a leave-in conditioner, hair vitamins, a moisturizer, and oil to your scalp. Then, tie braids with a satin scarf before bed.

Wigs

In order to enjoy wearing your wig, you must remember to protect your scalp and hair. When wearing any wig type, it is important to have the proper care program for your scalp hair and wig. There are many types of wigs to choose from, and wig makers are coming up with new ideas all the time. A few of the most common are toppers, integrations, falls, full-heads, and lace fronts, which come in both human and synthetic hair. I am often asked which types are safe and whether human or synthetic is better. Most wigs can be worn safely, but you will need to make some adjustments after you buy them.

When you purchase a wig, you must remember to make it hair-and scalp-safe. Start by turning the wig inside out, then removing any hooks, snaps, small combs, and any other little metal pieces from inside the wig. These things are used to hold your wig in place, but they are not hair- and scalp-friendly. These metal pieces can tear the hair and scalp, causing aging damage. Secure your wig using bobby pins.

The type of hair—human or synthetic—is up to you, and both can be worn safely. For full-head wigs you will need to wear a satin turban—not a stocking cap. The stocking cap keeps your natural hair tucked away; however, it pulls your hair because the band is much too tight at the hairline. I strongly recommend using a satin turban instead.

For many years there was one type of wig, and only celebrities could afford it. Now wig makers have made them affordable enough to be quite common among average consumers. Have you ever noticed how some celebrities' hair looks so natural you can't tell that they are wearing wigs? How their hairlines have baby-soft hair? We assume the hair must be natural, because at the part, we actually can see some scalp. Surprise! It's a hairpiece called a thin skin or, more commonly, a lace front wig. Lace fronts allow you to be free to wear any style, and you can comb and part the wig any way you want. This type of wig still costs a little more than the average store wig, but it is by far one of the most natural-looking of all wigs. The wig is sewn to a thin, lace-type fabric, which is then bonded to the entire hairline. A clear adhesive applied to the fabric allows you to have what appears to be an invisible hairline.

Many women create hair problems while wearing these wigs, because they do not remove it daily or even weekly. This is due, in part, to the fact that the manufacturer states that, if you remove the wig too often, it will cause unnecessary wear and tear to the hairpiece. As a result, many women will remove and reattach their wigs only once a month, which can cause their scalps and hair to become polluted. It is very important that you remove a lace front wig at least every two to three days in order to clean away pollutants and to condition your hair and scalp.

Wigs are worn by some women consistently and by others only occasionally. Wigs are convenient because they can be styled beforehand and then worn at times when you are rushed and don't have enough time to style your own hair. A number of celebrities even have their own lines of wigs that they market to the public. Other times, wigs are worn by women who are experiencing hair loss due to a number of health circumstances, generally, cancer patients who are going through chemotherapy or those who are suffering from alopecia. Added hair is something that can be enjoyed at any age and can help you look your best. Just remember the pros and cons and how to choose which one is right for you. So go ahead and enjoy wearing added hair without causing aging damage to your hair or scalp.

CHAPTER ELEVEN:

HOW CAN I PROTECT MY HAIR WHILE EXERCISING?

In this chapter, you will learn how to keep your hair from aging as you work out. You will also learn how to use the sauna and steam room to detoxify and condition the scalp and hair, which will help to protect the scalp and hair and prevent premature aging.

As we age, it becomes more and more apparent that our bodies could benefit from some type of workout program. Our doctors and all of the people who know and love us, as well as books, experts, and ads on television say in so many words that if you want to stay young and healthy, you must work out. We all agree that working out does help us feel better and look better as we age. But nowhere in any of those ads or in any conversations about working out, with any of those well-intentioned people is there any mention of what happens to our hair or what to do with our hair when we work out. Many women struggle with this, particularly black women. Some women struggle and feel forced to choose between working out and having great hair. I am here to tell you that you can do both. That is right: you can work out and have great hair. One of the challenges that women go through as they try to do both is, their hair tends to feel dry, look frizzy, and lack luster; the number one complaint is loss of style retention. A good cardio workout causes our body to overheat and sweat. You know what sweating does to a hairstyle: it causes the style to flop. So, often I hear from women, "My hair won't hold a style, and my scalp itches." But have you ever thought about why your hair won't hold a style and why your scalp itches? Or, more importantly, have you ever thought about what negative things sweat does to your hair and scalp?

Why Sweat?

As we all know, sweating is one of the body's ways of cooling itself off. It is an important natural process, because if we are not able to cool our bodies by sweating or some artificial method, such as pouring water on the body, our bodies could overheat, causing us to pass out. Sweating also helps to detoxify the body as it pushes waste and salt out of the skin's pores. Have you ever noticed how you feel after sweat dries on your body? You tend to feel sticky and dirty, and you can hardly wait to take a shower. Your hair and scalp go through changes when you work out.

If you work out and shower but don't shampoo your hair, your sweat will cause your hair and scalp to become dehydrated and polluted. After working out, even after a heavy cardiovascular session, many women will wait until their "regular shampoo day" to shampoo their hair. Some women will even have several workout sessions before shampooing their hair. The dry and dirty environment that you put your hair through and allow your hair and scalp to stay in will age your hair and scalp. Let's start with what happens to the scalp.

Remember that the scalp is skin, and just like the skin on your face, you must clean it on a regular basis, or you will develop a buildup in the pores. You have heard experts warn you about going to bed without washing away your makeup, because it can cause aging damage to your face. Well, your scalp has pores and follicles that must stay clear and clean in order to keep a healthy environment for healthy hair growth and to inhibit scalp problems, such as itchy scalp, or, worse, scalp disorders. When you sweat, your hair becomes dehydrated and brittle, and aging damage develops. This damage shortens the life of the strands. In order to maintain your hairstyle, while preventing your hair and scalp from aging as you enjoy your workout, you must have a plan of action. Working out is often a strain on our busy schedules, so it is hard to fit in time to restyle our hair. I believe we must find ways to create what I like to call a quick-fix hair and scalp care regimen. Now, when I say "quick-fix," it does not mean you should neglect to do certain things. If you have time to shower after a workout, you have time to do all that is necessary. By the time you finish your shower, you will have a clean and conditioned hair and scalp. One thing to remember is that you will be shampooing often, some weeks every day, so one application of a clarifying shampoo will be sufficient. Also, keep in mind that lots of rinsing is important.

Most workout programs have days that you do cardio, which causes you to sweat, and days you do weights, which may not cause you to sweat. One tip to remember is to shampoo on the days that you do your cardio workout; there is no need to shampoo your hair on the days you don't sweat.

Quick-Fix Part One: Clean and Condition

Step 1. In the shower, rinse your hair as you rinse your body.

Step 2. Apply shampoo to your hair and lather your body with it as well. Using an acid-balanced shampoo is safe on your hair, scalp, and body, and it saves time.

Step 3. Rinse your hair and body.

Step 4. Apply conditioner and let it sit while you shave your legs or lather your body one more time.

Step 5. Rinse your hair as you rinse your body.

You are now clean and conditioned from head to toe.

Part two of the quick-fix regimen is to style the hair, which for some can be a real challenge. When starting a workout program, some women will cut their hair short, get curly perms, or braid their hair with extensions. Those are options that you can choose, but don't ever feel forced. There are ways to keep your hair styled without making an atypical change just to manage your hair. Remember, you still need to keep your hair and scalp cleaned and conditioned. After your quick-fix shampoo and condition, you are ready for the next part.

Quick-Fix Part Two: The Five-Minute Hairstyle

Step 1. Wrap your head with a towel while you dry off.

Step 2. Remove the towel, and lightly apply a leave-in conditioner.

Step 3. Apply a sculptor setting lotion to your hairline. If your hair is curly, apply a moisturizer before the sculpting lotion, then smooth your hair back flat if it's short, or gather it into a ponytail using a cloth holder for longer hair.

Step 4. Spray a sculpting mist to your hair and hairline, and then tie a satin scarf around the hairline.

Step 5. Apply a hair attachment (e.g., bun, fall, or drawstring pony-tail).

Step 6. Secure the perimeter with bobby pins, and then remove the scarf.

There are many quick-fix styles that you can choose from. If you choose braids, remember that they are a low-maintenance style, but not a *zero*-maintenance style.

Saunas and Steam Rooms

Here's an idea to help you detoxify and condition your scalp and hair. Some women use the sauna and steam room when they visit the spa or after they work out. Besides being a relaxing treat, there are many benefits of the experience for your skin and hair.

Detoxification and Removal of Negative Buildup

Apply a clarifying shampoo to dry hair, massage it into the scalp, and rub down the strands. Now, place cotton around your hairline and put a plastic cap on your head. Sit for fifteen minutes or until you begin to sweat. While in the sauna, heat will help the clarifying shampoo to break down the buildup, making it easier to shampoo away all the various pollutants that collect on your hair and scalp.

Deep Conditioning

After shampooing your hair, towel-blot to remove excess water. Apply a liberal amount of conditioner to all strands. Next, cover your head with a plastic cap and then with a large towel. With the conditioner, you want deep penetration, but you don't want to sweat, so you should sit in the sauna for only three minutes. Be sure to drink 8 ounces of cold water to keep from sweating. Afterward, rinse your hair with warm water and apply a leave-in conditioner.

Deep Cleaning and Detoxification of Scalp Pores

Rinse your hair and scalp with warm water to remove the debris that may be sitting on top of your hair. Apply one application of clarifying shampoo and rub it throughout your hair. Rinse with warm water, and then blot away excess water. Reapply shampoo to your hair and scalp. Place cotton around your hairline, and cover your head with a plastic cap. Sit in the steam room for ten minutes. Afterward, rinse your hair and scalp thoroughly with very warm water. Apply one more application of clarifying shampoo, massage throughout, and rinse thoroughly for three minutes.

Things to Remember

- Avoid conditioning shampoos, because they will add buildup.
- Use a clarifying shampoo with a pH range between 4.5 and 5.5.
- Rinse with a strong water force.
- Use a moisturizing conditioner after detoxifying your hair.
- If you normally suffer from a dry scalp, remember to gently apply a small amount of leave-in, light oil on your scalp while it is still wet after rinsing and towel-blotting your hair.

The sauna and steam room can help detoxify your scalp and hair, as well as condition your hair, which is another enjoyable way to have a relaxing experience during your gym visit. Both prevent buildup and are good for deep conditioning, which will protect and preserve your hair and scalp and aid in the prevention of aging damage. You can enjoy your workouts and have great hair. Just remember to care for your hair and scalp's fitness as you care for your body's fitness. I understand the need to keep a style, but don't age your scalp and hair while achieving a younger body!

Chapter Twelve:

What Can I Do about Gray Hair?

In this chapter, you will learn how and why hair goes gray, as well as how to deal with and control this seemingly uncontrollable phenomenon. Also, you will learn how to keep your gray hair looking young.

Gray Hair

The combination of white and dark strands gives the illusion of gray or silver hair. When the dark hair is gone, all that is left is white. As melanocyte cells in the base of the hair follicle produce less and less melanin (color pigment), our hair will gradually lose the ability to produce any melanin within the affected follicle. The result is loss of hair color, leaving gray or white hair. The onset of this event is determined mostly by genetics. Even though some studies insist that stress, diet, and even certain environments will cause the hair to gray, researchers have found that there is little to nothing that you can do to stop your hair from turning gray. But don't let that stop you from looking for a way to stop your hair from graying! Just please be sure to share any findings with the rest of us. In the meantime, I have an answer for those of you who have a growing number of white fibers appearing each year, month, or seemingly every day.

Deal with it! This may not sound sympathetic, but I do mean just that: Deal with your gray hair, and do not let it deal with you, mentally or physically. In other words, don't think gray hair; think hair. Let's start with mental tribulations that occur when we go gray. We feel old. We think we look old. Next, let's look at the physical aspect. If we feel and think old, we dress and act old. Do you see where I am headed? This is no way to deal with gray hair; actually, it's letting your gray hair deal with you.

Dealing With It

Step one is to change your attitude and your approach toward your hair. Think about it: if you ever wanted to be a blond, now you are one! White hair is the blondest of blond, without the yellow. See, I made you smile. Step two is to choose whether or not to keep your hair gray. The rest is easy.

Make a choice. Do you want to color your gray hair? Then make a change. Or would you prefer to stay with white? Then learn the proper care for this new type of hair.

You may not have a choice in whether your hair turns gray, but you do have another choice. If you choose to cover your gray hair, make a conscious, well-informed decision and not some spur-of-the-moment, I-can't-take-it-anymore decision. Gray hair has dark hairs flowing between the white hairs, which have no color and act somewhat like a clean canvas. You can add whatever shade you like with little effort or risk of damage to the health of your hair and scalp. With dark hair, you must remove color pigments in order to change your hair color, which may require a strong peroxide-type chemical. With white hair, there is no color to remove, so you can bypass the damaging color-removing step. When choosing your color, do the research; you have certain considerations to take into account as well as options to choose from. I will share those options in detail in the next chapter on hair color.

Halo Hairline

Many have asked what to do about halo hairline. Halo hairline is that ring of white hair that seems just to appear only a week or so after coloring you hair. It is the line of demarcation where the color-treated hair ends and the white hair has begun to grow in again. The white hairline can be covered without going through the entire process of redoing your color each week. I recommend that you use a temporary brush-on color, one that will rinse away with each shampoo. Check your local wig or beauty supply stores; you can find brush-on colors in variations of brown, black, red, and blond. A very inexpensive and easy-to-use brush-on color, and one that many women use every day, is one you probably have in your makeup bag: that's right, mascara. It is important to avoid eye infections, so don't use the same mascara brush on your lashes that you will use on your hairline. Look for regular lash mascara, not waterproof mascara. The waterproof mascara contains a special wax that repels water and is harder to remove from the hair shaft; it will cause a buildup and make it difficult to condition and recolor the hairline areas. Mascara is safe, very inexpensive, easy to use, and you can find mascara in most of your local stores and supermarkets. But you will be limited to only black and brown shades.

One very important thing you must remember is that, even though all brush-on colors, including regular lash mascara, are safe to use on the hair, they are not scalp-friendly. When using any type of color, including rinses, spray-ons, and brush-ons, you must protect the scalp. If the color stains the scalp, it may become irritated and itchy. Over time, scalp pores will become clogged and, in extreme cases, temporary hairline balding could occur.

Stay Safe

Here is a simple routine to apply color safely. Looking in a mirror, part your hairline forward. Next, firmly hold the ends of the shaft and gently pull your hair straight with one hand while using your other hand to brush the color onto the white hairline, beginning with the hair closest to the scalp. This can be done every day and without ever touching the scalp.

Keep Your White Hair Looking Young

If you choose to keep your hair white and not add color, you need to have the proper care program, one that will give you youthful-looking hair. White hair tends to be somewhat uncontrollable; even the hairline hair will stick out as if it is on its own path. White hair also can start to look yellow or dull. In treating and consulting with women with white hair, I often hear them complain that their hair can be dry, coarse, lack luster, and stick out like wire. To keep your white hair clean, true to its natural white color, soft, shining, and shimmering, as well as manageable, you must have a plan to put into action.

Part A: Help Your Hair Keep Its Natural, White, Shimmering Glow

First, white hair will look dull if it is not cleaned with the proper shampoo and on a regular basis. Avoid shampoos that have red color additives, and stay away from conditioning shampoos. Red color additives can give your white hair a brassy tone. Conditioning shampoos will, over time, leave a film on your hair, giving it a dull look, lacking shine. Keep it simple: shampoo every three days with a clarifying shampoo, one that has the same pH as your hair (4.5 to 5.5).

Next, when using blow dryers and curling irons, keep the temperature on low to avoid burning the cuticle, or top layer, of the strand. When white hair is exposed to too much heat, it will yellow, indicating a burn on the shaft. Always use a leave-in conditioner—remember, no red or other dye additives.

Finally, be sure to shampoo after each time you are exposed to large amounts of smoke and dust for an extended period (e.g., conventions, parties, or outdoor events). Dust and smoke will leave a yellow cast on the hair shaft. To avoid this, use two applications of leave-in conditioner. Apply one application, wait sixty seconds, and then apply another application. It is a good idea to use a setting lotion before styling. Increasing the use of leave-in conditioners and setting products helps by placing a barrier between your hair and the components in the air. Remember to shampoo as needed to remove any pollutants.

Part B: Keep Your Hair Manageable and Under Control

First, to keep your hair under control, use a light cream moisturizer in place of mousse, gel, or other styling product. Be sure to stay away from any moisturizers that contain waxy ingredients, those that are any color other than white, and those whose first ingredient is water. Although some waxy-type moisturizers will seem to give you temporary control, these products tend to take away the body and bounce of your hair and leave it with a weighted-down look. Moisturizers that have color will slowly but eventually change the tint of your gray hair, causing a stained look. Nevertheless, moisturizers are a good idea because they help when your hair feels dry and brittle. Use a cream moisturizer, but not one that is too wet. It will give a damp, gel-like feeling when you apply it and will result in a fly-away, frizzy look. These things will only add to your problems and will not help you in your quest to get control of your gray hair.

To find the best moisturizer for you, I recommend that you go to your local beauty supply store and start reading the labels. Then, make a small investment and purchase the three most recommended hair moisturizers. Remember that you may find that the best ones actually are priced for less. There are many smaller manufacturers that have good products but cannot compete with larger companies' ads. When trying any new product on your hair, be sure your hair is clean and freshly conditioned. This will give you a true reading of how each moisturizer works with your hair. You want to look for a moisturizer that will leave your hair soft, but not so soft that your hairstyle does not hold. If you find a moisturizer that feels great, but your style doesn't seem to hold, try using less and less each time until you get the balance you want. I make and recommend Moisture Plus Moisturizer.

Second, if your hair is soft but lacks shine, be sure that all your hair products are water soluble, in other words, each one rinses clean. You should also use a shimmering shampoo for gray hair. Be sure to follow with a clarifying shampoo to avoid buildup.

Finally, you can lubricate your hair shaft using oil sheen in a jar. Lightly glaze your palms and, with open fingers, rub through dull areas only. You may need to adjust the amount depending on your hair texture: thin, fine, or naturally straight hair will need only half the amount needed for thick, coarse, or curly hair.

Chapter Thirteen:

What Do I Need to Know about Hair Coloring?

In this chapter, you will learn about hair color categories and changing your hair color. You will understand how each category of hair color differs and how to prevent hair and scalp aging when choosing from amongst them. Also, I'll tell you how to achieve a healthy shine as well as the youthful look of radiance for your natural hair color if you decide not to color your hair.

No one has to walk around on this earth with gray hair, and as we age, we may want to cover our gray hair, and sometimes we want to change our hair color completely just for something different. I strongly believe that choosing to change your hair color is a beautiful way for you to express yourself. Unfortunately, many women end up with the wrong color or a color that they didn't want. To prevent this from happening to you, there are things that you must know about hair color before choosing to change yours.

As we age, our natural hair color can change, sometimes slightly, sometimes completely. This could be a problem when choosing hair color. You may have used a particular color for years and gotten the same satisfying results, but decided to stop coloring your hair for a while. However, when you decided to resume coloring your hair and went back to that same color, the results were different. You may have questioned the company and thought that it changed the formula. More likely, it wasn't the color in the bottle that changed; it was your natural hair color that changed. Throughout our lives we experience a change in hair pigments, and this change will cause variations in color when we color treat our hair. When hair is color treated we are doing one of two things. We are either depositing pigments into or removing pigments from our hair. If your hair is light and you want to darken it, the process will be to deposit pigments into the hair. If your hair is dark and you want to lighten it, then the process will be to remove pigments.

Choosing a Color

Many women want to express themselves with a change of hair color but may be afraid for a variety reasons:

- They worry that it will be the wrong color.
- They are nervous that it won't look right on them.
- They are concerned that it won't match their skin tone.
- They wonder what people will say.
- They fear that it might damage their hair.

The list could goes on and on. Many have asked, "How do I know which color is right for me?" I am a strong believer in seeking professional advice and opinions before having a color applied. But I am equally strong in my belief that you must choose a shade that you feel comfortable wearing. I am sure all the colorists at this point, are not happy with me. Quite simply, the color that is right for you is the one that gives you that feeling when you look in the mirror and say, "This is right."

I believe that, as we grow older, we should also have some fun, even if it means becoming somewhat of a daredevil. However, you must be careful, because you can't safely color your hair over and over, trying to find the right color. This eventually will cause aging damage to your hair and scalp. If you have been thinking about a certain color, and everyone—even professionals—says that it is all wrong for you, I have a simple, fun, and safe suggestion.

First, choose a day when you have a generous amount of free time, preferably a day during the middle of the week when stores are not as busy. Go to a wig store and buy a wig the color you are thinking about. It is very important that you choose a wig that matches the texture and type of your hair. You also may find it helpful to have the wig cut in the same style as your hair. Put on the wig and look in the mirror at the person looking back at you. Notice how you feel about the way you look. Now put the wig—and your new color—to the test: wear it for your family around the house, for your friends when you get together, to work, to the supermarket, wherever you go. Give yourself about a week of parading around, then make your own decision about whether this color is right for you. Keep trying with as many wigs and colors as it takes until you find the right shade. This is a small investment to make, and it will be worth it because it will save your hair and scalp from the damage that occurs when your hair is colored too often.

After choosing a hair color, I highly recommend that you seek the help of a colorist. Some things should be left to the professional. You can wear your wig and say to your colorist, "Make me look like this." Your colorist will be able to assist you in getting the tones just right for your skin. But don't let her talk you into changing the shade too much. Stay assertive, don't be excluded, and the end result will be one that you feel happy with.

Hair Color Categories

Hair color comes in three categories: temporary, semipermanent, and permanent. It is important that you understand how each category differs, as well as how your hair and scalp will respond to the application of each category. A lack of understanding of color categories and each type within that particular category, as well as of application and maintenance, will lead to aging damage of your strands, even shortening their lives.

Temporary Hair Colors

Temporary hair colors are considered nonchemical. They contain topical colors that are safe to use at home and remain on the hair only from one shampoo until the next. This category has very little chance of causing aging damage because they contain mostly water with a substance that temporarily coats the hair, similar to a conditioner. There are other types of temporary hair colors that can be sprayed on, drawn on, or even rubbed on, but these contain wax and require a remover that is made for each particular color. Temporary colors are not as popular as the other two categories of colors because they offer very little change to your natural color. However, there are some women who like them for precisely that reason, and because they are an easy introduction to experimenting with new colors. So allow me to explain the two most popular types of temporary hair colors.

Temporary color rinses

Temporary color rinses are also known as shampoo-in/shampoo-out colors. They are nonchemical and safe to use weekly. These rinses work by coating the hair strand, but they cannot change or add color to dark hair. Temporary colors take your existing color and change it slightly. They have no ability to deposit color to the cuticle, nor do they have the ability to stain the cuticle layer. These rinses are most often used on light or gray hair, slightly altering your hair, ridding it of that dull, yellow look.

You can purchase temporary colors at your local beauty supply stores and even some discount stores. The consistency of a temporary color rinse is similar to water, and the color lasts only until the next shampoo. After your hair has been shampooed and conditioned, towel-blot to dry your hair and then apply the color to hair. Finish with leave-in conditioners and styling products.

Color shampoo

A color shampoo is nonchemical and should not be mistaken for a shampoo-in color, which is a chemical. Because of the twist of words, many women get the two confused. Color shampoo is a shampoo combined with color rinses. These temporary enhancers create very little, if any, noticeable color change on dark hair, but they do provide a slight highlight for lighter hair. They can be purchased at your local beauty supply store.

Semipermanent Colors

A semipermanent color, better known as a rinse, can deposit color on or stain the cuticle of the hair strand, as well as highlight or cover old, dull, previously tinted hair. Because semipermanent colors can only deposit artificial color on your cuticle layers, there will be no real lightening of your hair. Many women with dark hair believe that if they use a light brown or blond rinse, their hair actually will become light brown or blond. When the desired results are not achieved, they just don't understand why, and they are very disappointed and sometimes angry with their stylists. It is important to understand that a rinse used on dark hair may not offer any apparent color change. In cases where the hair color is light, however, you can see a slight to very noticeable highlighting.

Semipermanent color should be applied only to clean, wet hair directly after it has been shampooed and conditioned. This type of color can remain on the cuticle for as little as one week or as long as six months, and in some cases longer depending on the porosity of the hair. Semipermanent colors can have drying and aging effects on the hair and scalp if the color is not rinsed completely or if the hair is not thoroughly conditioned before and after the application. However, if used properly, this category of hair coloring is safe to use at home and can be purchased at your local beauty supply stores. If you don't have a clear understanding of or are not sure how to apply the color, I always recommend that you seek the help of a colorist, someone who is an expert and can help you decide what is best for your hair.

As I mentioned earlier, semipermanent colors will either stain the cuticle layer or deposit color into the cuticle layers. For your benefit, I will describe each type and let you know which one I recommend.

Stain semipermanent color rinses

These will stain the cuticle layer with artificial pigments for one week or many months, depending on how porous your hair is. The stain rinses such as black or dark brown are used mostly to cover gray hair. You can also find stain rinses in many tones of red, brown, and even blond, which are used to highlight gray or your naturally lighter shades that you may have throughout your hair. This is why some stain rinses, when applied, will leave strong red tones that look grape-red or even purple-red. And some black stain rinses will leave strong blue-black tones. In a quest to get their hair as black as possible, as well as in hopes to make the black "hold," many African American women will request blue-black colors specifically.

The frustration with using a stain rinse is that it is very messy to apply and does not last very long. Sometimes clients will request applications every week, because in some cases the color will rinse away after each shampoo. Another annoyance is that the stain rinse can bleed onto your pillow case as well as onto your collar when you sweat. How embarrassing is that? However, the real problem with this type of rinse is that, if used over a period of time, it can cause damage to both the hair and the scalp. Stain rinses do not rinse clean from the hair; they leave traces of color that extremely dehydrate the shaft, making the hair look dull and feel brittle. This dehydration will damage the shaft, causing the cuticle layers to lift, and ultimately thin your strands. When using a stain rinse, you may notice that your scalp is also colored. This is very dangerous because that scalp stain is actually color residue that did not rinse clean. This residue can clog your scalp pores, which includes the mouth of the hair follicle. Also, it will dehydrate the scalp, causing scalp itch; scratching your scalp begins the process of aging damage. Needless to say, this type of semipermanent rinse is not a good choice, and I would go so far as to highly recommend that you stay away from all rinses that stain and dry out your scalp and hair.

Deposit semipermanent color rinses

These will deposit artificial pigments into the cuticle layers of the strand. This type of rinse is safe and will not cause any aging damage to your hair when used properly. Make sure your hair is well conditioned beforehand and reconditioned thoroughly after the color is rinsed, and your hair and scalp will fare well. Deposit semipermanent color rinses are mixed with solutions that allow the cuticle layers to accept the color, literally becoming part of the cuticle layers. This type of rinse fades very slowly, which gives an almost permanent effect to the hair shaft. Since the cuticle layers are transparent, having no color, the deposited tones pick up and reflect light. This is why when you are in a room with low lighting it is hard to see your semipermanent color. The more light your hair is exposed to, the more you can see the color, especially when exposed to natural sunlight.

Deposited semipermanent rinses come in shades of black, which deposits a deep, dark oriental black tone to hair; and dark brown, which deposits a brown tone to the hair that shows up as dark brown on lighter hair or as a deeper, more even brown on dark hair. Some clients expect to see more of the brown color, and many times they are not happy with the finished color; some will even say that their hair seemed darker before the rinse was applied. The reason the color does not seem noticeably darker is that with most white and black women their dark hair has variations of medium brown tones in their natural color. When a deposit rinse is applied, it will even out everything into a dark brown color. Red dyes deposit red tones to the hair in various degrees, depending on how light the hair originally is. There are some basic shades that may vary within their particular color in order to give a variety of effects as the tones reflect light.

Deposit semipermanent color rinses are safe to use at home, but I recommend that you seek the help of a colorist, one who has experience with these rinses. This will help to avoid the frustration of choosing the wrong color, and also will prevent aging damage to the hair and scalp. Be aware of two things when choosing rinses. First, dark stain or deposited black rinses will become permanent if your hair is overly porous. If you want the color removed, it will need to be stripped away.

This stripping process may leave your hair dry, which will cause aging damage to your hair. Second, you must choose one that rinses clean, and you must have a good shampooing and conditioning regimen in order to prevent aging your hair and scalp.

Permanent hair colors

Permanent color is a lasting chemical change to the hair shaft. The process involves either depositing pigments into or removing pigments from the cortex layer of the shaft. The cortex layer lies within the strand, resting next to the cuticle layer, and is the part of the strand that houses the pigments that give your hair its natural color. Permanent colors, unlike semipermanent colors, can completely change your natural color to very light shades or to very dark shades. Furthermore, they last until that strand is cut, sheds away, or is changed to a new color.

In order to lighten your dark hair, the process removes pigment. The chemical is applied to the hair and travels through the cuticle layers into the cortex layers. Next, the chemical begins lifting or removing your natural pigments until a lighter shade is achieved. The finished color will be dependent on the original color of your hair, the porosity of your hair, and the color of the tone that was applied. For example, if your hair is black, and you apply a blond tint, the result will not be a blond head of hair. The reason is that the basic OTC lighter color choices are tint chemical colors, which will remove only about three shades of color. This means your previously black hair will end up somewhere in the red family. A colorist can offer professional color products that will give you the desired shade.

In order to take your light hair to a dark shade, the process involves depositing artificial color pigments. The chemical passes through the cuticle layers and deposits variations of these dark pigments into the cortex layer.

I want to emphasize a point of safety for you. Even though this is a chemical change to your hair, and even though the color is called permanent, it does not have to be an irreversible change. You can choose to change your hair from light to dark and back to light, but be aware that each time this is done the hair goes through a traumatic experience. The process is traumatic because it affects the two main layers: the cuticle and the cortex. If these layers are harmed, aging damage will occur throughout the entire strand. Your hair will become lifeless, dry, and brittle and can even break, shortening the life of your strands. There are many choices of permanent hair coloring, from tints to bleaching, to achieve lowlights or highlights. It is important to remember that all are categorized as a chemical process. I highly recommend that you seek a professional who specializes in the application of permanent hair color and who is knowledgeable about the care of the hair and scalp during and after the process.

Have a Youthful Look of Radiance with Your Natural Hair Color

You don't have to change your own natural color to have youthful, radiant hair. All your hair needs to have a healthy shine is healthy cuticles; light reflects off healthy hair cuticles. The cuticle layer is the layer of your strand that takes the most abuse, because it is very exposed, resting on the outside of the strand. You must work to preserve these protective layers in order to have a youthful shine with your natural hair color. Avoid high temperatures when using heated tools. Be careful with bristle brushes, and never roughly comb your hair. You should also lubricate the hair cuticles when in a dry environment by rubbing oil on curly or dry hair or by glazing oil on straight or thin hair. But be sure that the oil rinses clean from your hair with each shampoo. Otherwise, your hair will develop a negative buildup, causing a dull appearance that defeats the purpose. Your natural color can be even more beautiful than any added color if you follow tips I have mentioned.

Are There Youthful Hair Colors and Styles?

In this section you will learn how the wrong choice in style, color, or cut can make you look older. I will help you to choose the style, cut, and color that will take years off your face. I feel that it is important to have a stylist, and maybe even a makeup expert, to assist you with your hair color and styles. I want to aid in empowering you so that you can stay assertive when choosing and talking to the various experts. Therefore, I will give you some suggestions and advice.

We have talked about the importance of understanding the various types of hair color and the effect that each type has on your hair. It is also important as we think about rinses and styles as we age that we understand and recognize which choice of style and color will cause us to look older. This is what I call a style issue. Before I entered the trichology field, I worked as a hairstylist for more than ten years, and my forte was hair designing. I could create just the right hairstyle and color combination for my clients. I became astute at noticing that certain colors, styles, and tools could make a client's hair or face look aged. I never wanted a client to be dissatisfied with my work, so I was careful always to do whatever was needed to make a perfect fit. Have you every received a certain color and immediately felt you looked older or felt your hair looked dull and drab? When you choose a color, you must be sure it will compliment your skin tone and face shape. Let me share some tips with you.

Tips

The general rule of thumb is: the lighter your skin, the lighter your hair color; the darker your skin, the darker your hair color. The trick to wearing lighter colored hair if you have dark skin is to highlight your hair. If your skin is light in tone, then lowlight some of your hair to get a darker color. However, you must have everything in the correct proportion, or you will create a disaster. For dark skin you want to have most of the hair that is closest to your face dark, with a few highlights blended in. For light skin you want to have most of the hair closest to your face light, with a few lowlights blended in. This will give your skin a lift, and it will prevent that washed out, drab look.

Make sure your highlights and lowlights are complimentary to your face shape and are appropriate for your skin's age (e.g., do you have wrinkles?). Your goal should be to create more of a pear shape to your face, because it is the most youthful of all face shapes. The right color combination can help also to minimize the appearance of lines and wrinkles; you and your stylist should spend some time discussing how to deemphasize them.

Let's create a hypothetical situation to sum up these tips. Suppose you have a round face shape and dark skin. Add some highlights around the sides of your face. Suppose you have a round-shaped face with light skin. Add a few lowlights around your face to make your face appear more youthful with a pear shape. If you have lines and wrinkles, you never want to draw attention to them! As I said before, I recommend that you contact a stylist, colorist, and maybe even a makeup expert to help you select the perfect style and color.

CHAPTER FOURTEEN:

WHAT IF I WANT TO STRAIGHTEN OR CURL MY HAIR?

In this chapter you will learn about temporary curly and temporary straight style options. Also, you will learn about the permanent changes that occur within the hair. I will explain the chemical changes that occur during a permanent wave or permanent straighter. Finally, you will learn how to create them while preventing aging damage to your hair.

Temporary Curly and Temporary Straight Style Options

As women, we really take the phase "it's my prerogative" to the limits, especially when it comes to our hair and how we style it. There are many things that women don't like about their hair, but the number one thing on the list is the shape of the strand. Some of us are born with curly and some with straight hair, and both are happy, but we must admit that many women just are not pleased with the crown of tresses that they have been blessed with. I have listened to women boldly say,

"I just don't like my hair," and some go as far as to say, "I hate my hair!" If their hair is naturally curly, then they want it straight; and if their hair is naturally straight, then they want it curly. And sometimes we just don't know which we want. We spend weeks with a curly look, then switch to straight hair, and then fluctuate almost daily, trying out different variations of straight and curly looks!

Oh yes, we have a ball with our hair, and we justify what seems to be an uncertainty about how we want to look by saying, "I will do whatever I want with my hair, and I don't care what anyone thinks because I am comfortable in my own skin." I love this newfound attitude that we develop as we age, but as it relates to our hair we must be careful when we express ourselves. Keep in mind that each one of your hair strands has only one life, and you don't want to shorten it. Therefore, we must learn about temporary curly and temporary straight style options and how to safely achieve them, preventing aging damage to our hair and scalp.

When you think of creating a straight or curly look temporarily, what do you think is needed to achieve this? Most commonly women turn to some form of heat. The heated tools of choice for women with curly hair are usually flat irons, curling irons, and pressing combs. Women with straight hair tend to use curling irons, crimping irons or heat rollers. Also, one must not forget everyone's favorite: the blow dryer. Women with all types of hair typically start the styling torture with a blow dryer. I call it torture because heated tools are almost always overused. One day after examining the hair of a particular patient, I told her that her strands had heat damage, which was causing her to lose hair. She was shocked and said, "That is impossible! I don't curl my hair every day. I only use the curling iron occasionally, so I am sure you must be mistaken." My response to her was "That is the same thing the lady said to the doctor when he told her she was pregnant." It is not how often you do something; it is about what happens *when* you do it. You can use heated tools without causing aging damage if you understand one simple thing: Your hair strands can tolerate only a certain amount of heat, about 250 to 300 degrees, and that is on healthy strands, and then the strand must be allowed to cool down completely. When your hair is overheated (exposed to more than 300 degrees), the layers will begin to expand, lift, then melt away. This results in aging damage that will lead to hair loss.

Over-processing with a Heated Styling Tool

Heated tools are some of the most popular styling aids and are used to temporarily straighten or curl hair. Curling irons, spiral wands, pressing combs, and flat irons are considered pressured heat. Unfortunately, thousands of women suffer from aging damage because of direct-pressure heat from these styling tools. You may have heard that a chemical can over-process your hair, but you may not have known that a heated tool also can over-process your hair. I am not saying that a heated tool will cause instant breakage. Over-processing from a heated tool is more like a slow death to your strands. The temporary style is achieved by high levels of pressure heat applied to the hair strand. The cuticle layers melt away as the bands within the cortical fibers become damaged. Over time this melting away of the top protective layers from this pressured heat causes the remaining fiber to become thin and permanently straight and weak.

Hair Strand Damage

If you have curly hair, you may have noticed that after pressing your hair for a while, your hair began to change. Your hair became thin, and when you shampooed, your hair did not return to its natural curly state. It was as if part of your strands had been relaxed. This is a clear sign that your hair has been over-processed.

If you have straight hair, you may have noticed that your hair became thin and lost volume and fullness. You may have noticed also that your hair didn't hold a curl, no matter how small of a curling iron you used. Each time your hair strands are exposed to more heat than they can tolerate, the top protective layers melt away little by little, the cortex becomes exposed, and the actual strand size becomes smaller as the bonds within the cortex become completely flattened.

Scalp Damage

I also want to make you aware of the potential for scalp damage from heated tools. I am sure you can recall instances when you, or even your stylist, got a little too close and accidentally touched your scalp with a heated tool. You were fully aware of the terrible pain you felt as the heat burned your skin, but you may not have been aware of the aging damage that resulted from that painful experience. Sometimes when your scalp and hair are overexposed to heat, they seem just to bounce back.

But it is not a bouncing back experience that occurs! It is more of a wearing down consequence. When this type of damage takes place repeatedly, the life of each of your strands is shortened, and your hair thins then breaks away. Your scalp even may lose its ability to produce new strands; in other words, balding will occur as a result of scarring.

Rules for Safely Using Heated Styling Tools

You don't have to give up your heated tools, but when you do use them you will need to follow some strict rules that will prevent aging damage to your hair and scalp.

1. Monitor the heat by using an oven thermometer, which you can pick up at any grocery store. Simply place the heated tool on the metal portion of the thermometer Remember you want to use less than 300 degrees; I recommend about 150 to 250 degrees.

2. Use heated tools only on clean hair. Dirty hair burns easily.

3. Always use a leave-in conditioner (e.g., moisturizer for curly that is natural or chemically relaxed; spray-on conditioner for naturally straight hair).

4. Remove heat rollers before they cool; allow a maximum of three minutes for each section of hair. Overheating the hair with rollers could create tears along the layers of the strand.

5. Never turn on heated tools until you are ready to use them. Most curling irons and flat irons will begin to overheat after they have been sitting for a while.

6. Try using indirect heat, such as a wet setting, and then sit under the dryer.

Burning your hair and scalp with heated tools can cause the development of the disorders Short Hair Syndrome (SHS) and Follicular Epidermis Alopecia (FEA), which I discussed in Chapter Six. There you learned more techniques and tools that offer safe ways to create both curly and straight looks without damaging your hair and scalp.

Permanent Curly and Permanent Straight Style Options

Most women use the term *perm* when referring to either when the hair is permanently waved or permanently straightened. A perm can give you what seems to be the ultimate control or style manageability over your hair. A perm chemically and permanently removes or adds curl to the hair during one life or hair growth cycle. Women of all nationalities and with all types of hair believe that a perm is an answer to their prayers, until hair loss and scalp damage occur. As a result, women are likely to have a love-hate relationship with perms.

There are many different reasons why women have these up-and-down feelings. But all of the reasons stem from the lack of full understanding of what a perm is. Although most women have a vague idea that a chemical is applied to their hair, women are in the dark about the serious changes that occur and the potential damage to the hair when it is permanently relaxed or curled. They also lack knowledge of what physical harm these chemicals can cause to the hair and scalp. Chemical damage is one of the leading causes of hair loss among women in America and some other parts of the world. Pay close attention to the things I explain for you here before you choose to chemically treat your hair. The knowledge you gain will empower you to prevent aging damage to your hair and scalp and may just save your hair's life.

Kitchenticians

Thousands of women go to local beauty stores to purchase home perm kits and do perms for themselves, their daughters, and their friends. I call them kitchenticians. These women are led to believe that all they need to do is read the label on the box and they'll be armed and equipped to perform a chemical treatment that, in reality, should be performed only by a licensed professional. But remember, this licensed professional must be trained in the pretreatment of the hair before a perm as well as the application and maintenance of a permanent chemical service.

The Chemical Change

When a chemical relaxer or wave is applied to your hair, many changes occur within the hair strand. The cuticle (top layer) opens to allow the chemical to pass through to the cortex (second layer), where the chemical change actually occurs. In short, the chemical rearranges delicate bonds within the cortex in order to permanently change the structure (shape) of your strands.

Issues That Women Face with a Permanent Relaxer

Women of all nationalities have curly hair, varying in degree from a slight wave to an extremely tight corkscrew. The label "hard to manage" definitely describes this type of hair. Women with curly hair struggle to slide a comb straight through, without a yanking and pulling tug-of-war. Many women, for whatever reason, believe that their hair is more manageable and better groomed when the curl is removed from the strand.

I believe that such thoughts as those have indirectly caused much damage to the hair of curly-haired women. I feel strongly that if we learn to accept, manage, and love our hair in its natural state, whether it is curly or straight, we would suffer less from aging damage. Although it may sound like I am contradicting myself, I equally believe that a woman has the right to chemically treat her hair and wear it very curly, slightly wavy, or straight. What I take issue with is the unnecessary harm, which shortens the life of the strand, that seems inevitably to go along with using chemicals. I have made it one of my missions in life to change the thoughtless, careless use of chemicals that leads to destructive aging damage.

There are many women who desire to straighten their spiral locks, and they have searched far and wide for any solution. The most popular one is a chemical relaxer. The relaxer business is big, and the manufacturers spend tons of money to market their product via radio, TV, and magazine ads as they parade beautiful models with that straight, shining, perfect hair. What you do not see in those ads is the high percentage of women who suffer from aging damage to their hair and scalp from relaxers. It is important to understand the process of relaxing hair.

First, the relaxer softens some of the curly pattern. Next, as the process continues, the relaxer begins to change the hair into a permanent straight form. If the relaxer is left on the hair any longer than is needed to complete the straightening process, the relaxer will cause the strands to become thin and weak. If left on even longer, it will continue to break down the strands until your hair is so thin and weak that it reaches its final threshold, at which point the hair will dissolve and die. The damage is that simple: when a relaxer is done improperly or repeated too soon, you run the risk of hair loss.

The fact is most women who use relaxers deal with a certain level of chemical damage at one point or another, and this has driven some women with curly hair back to their "natural roots." A rapidly growing percentage of black women are going back to their true head of hair. Many black women literally run away in fear from relaxers because of the scalp problems and hair loss that they experience. These problems stem from the aging damage that is a result of the misuse and overuse of the chemicals used to relax curls.

Also bearing weight is the fact that, after relaxing their hair, many black women act as if their hair were healthy and naturally straight. This is problematic because the needs of healthy, naturally straight hair are very different from chemically straightened hair. The hair goes through a transformation from curly to straight that is very traumatic for your hair and scalp, leaving your hair vulnerable and out of balance. In order to protect and preserve your hair and scalp and prevent aging damage, it is important that you have a hair and scalp care regimen that includes deep conditioning.

Black women have issues with chemical relaxers that are specific to them and that have caused an extreme amount of hair loss. One issue in particular stems from the belief that if they don't get a touch-up at the first sign of new growth, the hair will break. Many professionals also believe and tell their clients this. I totally disagree; my studies have shown that women who relax their hair immediately at the sign of new growth suffer from aging damage. I have concluded that a large percentage of black women have what appears to be a relaxer addiction. Yes, a relaxer is, for many black women, their hair drug of choice. Every month they must have their relaxer fix, or they panic. Well, the truth is the lack of manageability of the new growth is what causes them to rush out for a touch-up.

I would like to share with you some of the other things that I discovered in my studies. The line where the newly grown natural hair ends and the chemically treated hair begins is the line of demarcation, or as I like to put it, the line of difference. At that line, a sort of war begins. Let me draw you a clear picture: Curly hair swirls from your scalp and takes on a C shape; however, as it grows to about a half-inch, the hair acquires a full S or spiral shape. As the new hair continues to grow in, these thousands of spiral fibers begin to cross over each other. As the natural hair grows farther away from the scalp, it can become tangled and even matted to the scalp area. Many women will fix that by having their stylist apply more relaxer. The danger is that the scalp can become overexposed, and the hair can become over-processed, causing the epidermal scalp layers to become thin. The average black women has a relaxer applied somewhere between every four to six weeks.

Erroneously, the manufacturers of these chemicals say that it is safe to use them every six weeks. But the average strand is growing only about half an inch every five to eight weeks—not nearly enough growth to require nor justify a touch up. Moreover, studies have shown that as we age our hair grows slower, so it is growing at a rate closer to half an inch every eight weeks; some of the hair may be growing even slower, depending on genetics.

My point is, if you have your hair relaxed every four to six weeks, you will have only about a half-inch of new growth for your stylist to work with. Without enough new growth, your stylist will overlap the chemical onto the previously relaxed hair, and because a relaxer causes a permanent change to the hair, the hair will become over-processed. This ages and thins the hair, ultimately causing hair loss.

Issues That Women Face with a Permanent Wave

There are no degrees of straightness to straight hair. At the first sign of a small ripple, the strands are no longer considered straight; they are considered curly or wavy. Many women with straight hair want curly hair, and oftentimes in their quest to achieve this, they turn to chemicals to create permanent waves or curls. The degree of curl that women want will vary with the reason for the added curl. You may want to have a tight curly perm with hopes that it will be easy to wash and wear, saving you time. There are two problems with this line of thinking. First, a lot of women believe that a curly perm is a no-maintenance style, when in fact a curly perm is a low-maintenance style. Second, all tight curly perms cause some level of over-processed aging damage to the strands. Remember that the need for deep conditioning to preserve your strands is even greater after the curly perm. Unfortunately, many women just won't take the time to do that.

How to Prevent Aging Damage When Getting a Perm

The permanent changes that occur within the hair when you receive a permanent wave can be achieved without damaging the hair and scalp. For chemical perm services, you need a professional who will help to determine the best application and chemicals that will allow you to safely achieve your desired style. A hair and scalp analysis should be done to determine whether they are in a healthy state. The analysis should be preformed by a trichologist, who examines your hair and scalp using a handheld microscope with various magnification lenses. These lenses allow the trichologist to view the scalp, see the condition of the epidermal layers and the strand, and see the condition of the hair cuticles. This type of examination is invaluable because it will give you the information you need to avoid scalp burns and hair loss. Additionally, this examination not only will expose any damage that may be present, but it also will reveal your natural hair type, its elasticity and porosity, and the multiple hair textures throughout your hair.

Elasticity is the ability of the hair strand to stretch and expand without breaking. Good elasticity is important because a certain amount of swelling and stretching occurs during a chemical process. Porosity determines how the hair will absorb the chemical. Good porosity also is important because it will ensure that your hair will process the chemical in a controlled manner, giving the best possible results.

You should request a full report of your analysis; a small fee may be attached to this request, but it will be worth it. Give your hair stylist a copy. The information in this report will aid your stylist in determining the proper steps for preparing your hair and scalp for the chemical service. When I perform a hair and scalp analysis, I allow and even recommend that the stylist sit in during the examination. I also offer my clients free counseling by phone, in which I discuss the details of their analysis with their stylist in cases when the stylist is not available at the time of the examination.

Simple Rules to Follow Before a Chemical Service

1. Have a hair and scalp analysis before any type of chemical service.
2. Never chemically treat hair that is damaged.
3. Always have the chemical process done by an expert who specializes in the type of service that you want to receive. It is important that the expert is someone with experience working with your hair type and texture.
4. Never have permanent chemical relaxer or curl treatment applied to hair that has been previously chemically treated. Remember, because most chemical processes are permanent, touching up or repeating the service on the previously chemically treated portion of the hair strand will cause over-processing and lead to aging damage.

5. Only chemically treat the natural portion of the strand (the hair closest to the scalp).
6. Always follow a strict maintenance care program.

Anyone can avoid the damage that occurs when a chemical is applied if she understands the chemical changes that occur. The ability to have straight or curly hair, whether temporarily or permanently, can be achieved and enjoyed without aging damage. Just remember to stay within these guidelines and follow the rules.

INDEX

aged, 16
aging. See Aging
breakage, 2. See also Breakage
bulb, 36, 41
club, 36
coarse, 66
depression, x
drying, 63–64
end, 14, 15
follicle. See Follicle
gray, 129–135
growth cycle, 12, 14, 32–37
infusion, 113
pH of, 60
porosity, 61–62
regrowth, 73
replacement techniques, 75
scalp, 14, 19–20. See also Scalp
shaft. See Shaft
shape, 30. See also Type
strand. See Strand
thinning, xii. See also Thinning hair
white, 132–135
Hair Doctor, the, 165
Hair loss
and age, 70
alopecia areata, 75–76
and behavior, 77–79
categories of, 70
external follicle, 70, 76–79, 81
female pattern baldness, 74–75, 81
internal follicle, 45, 70–76
myths, 67–70
natural, 36–37. See also Shedding
permanent, 34
preventing, 49–52
and scratching, 58
treating, 43–44
women, 7
Hair Nutrition System, 165
Hairpieces, 75, 105–106
Hairstyles
five-minute, 124–125
tips for, 149–150

Halo hairlines, 131–132
Health conditions, 72
Heat, 64–65, 83, 153–154
Hormones, 45, 72, 74
Hypodermis, 20–21, 25–26

I

Illness, severe, 72
Internet, the, 39
Itch, 20, 57–59

K

Kitchenicians, 157

L

Lace fronts, 118
Layer
peeling, 41
preserving, 147
strand, 60

M

Maintenance, 106–109
Mascara, 131–132
Massage, 92
Medication, 47–48, 72
Medicine, 41–42
Medulla, 28
Men
behavior of, 81
spending by, ix
Menopause, 11–12, 70–71, 74
Minoxidil, 74
Moisturizer, 66
buying, 134–135
for white hair, 134

ABOUT THE AUTHOR

Hair guru **Lisa Akbari**, also known by her patients as "The Hair Doctor," started in the beauty and hair care field over thirty years ago as a licensed cosmetologist and aesthetician, and is now a board certified Trichologist. Through her seminars, workshops, classes, and books, the "Hair Doctor" educates patients, dermatologists, and hairstylists on how to prevent aging hair. Akbari along with her husband, Hooshang Akbari, are the directors and lead Trichologists of Hair Nutrition and Research in Memphis Tennessee, which focuses on education, research, and analysis of hair and its connection to the scalp. Akbari has authored two books: *The Journey from Kinky to Straight (and All Its Pitstops)*, and *The Black Woman's Guide to Beautiful Hair*, which is the number-one selling hair care book on the market today. Akbari has developed and now manufactures a full line of hair treatment and maintenance products called the Hair Nutrition System. Akbari has been featured on a number of radio talk shows as well as in newspapers and magazines, including *Jet* and *Grace*. She directs the Trichology Program at Southwest Community College in Memphis, Tennessee.

Visit the "Hair Doctor" at the Healthy Hair Group, her virtual salon, at www.lisaakbari.com.